Autism.
A Quick Immersion

*Quick Immersions* provide illuminating introductions to diverse topics in the worlds of social science, the hard sciences, philosophy and humanities. Written in clear and straightforward language by prestigious authors, the texts also offer valuable insights to readers seeking a deeper knowledge of those fields.

Maria J. Portella

# AUTISM
## A Quick Immersion

Tibidabo Publishing
New York

Translated by Lori Gerson
Cover art by Raimon Guirado

First published: October 2022

Visit our Series on our Web:
www.quickimmersions.com

ISBN: 978-1-949845-34-1
1 2 3 4 5 6 7 8 9 10

Library of Congress Control Number: 2022940092

Printed in the United States of America.

To Roger and Jordi (I love you so much)

# Acknowledgments

When I published my first book *Mundos Invisibles: The Autism Spectrum explicado por una madre neurocientífica* (Invisible Worlds, the autism spectrum explained by a neuroscientist mother), I never thought that within three years I would write another. Having Antoni Comas as an editor makes everything possible, and here I am. Thus, my first thanks goes to my editor (how I love saying I have an editor) and the team at Tibidabo Publishing.

The lockdown and being able to work from home, following the outbreak of COVID-19, gave me a unique opportunity to write about autism. Because without realizing it, I once again had the need to share everything I had been learning over the last three years by giving talks and having workshops and encounters with the brave, wonderful people in the autism associations all throughout Catalonia and in other psychiatric services for children and young people. Thank you for sharing so much knowledge!

Joan Trujols and Àngela Vidal have been my first readers on this occasion. Their contributions have permeated some of the fundamental sections of this book with humanity and respect, and for this I am extremely grateful to them. They have also been critical of the data and information I have expressed, and their corrections have given the work a higher quality. Thank you so much!

Thanks to all of you, friends and family, who are always there (also to you, Rafel, whom I always carry in my heart).

Finally, I want to thank Jordi, my husband, and Roger, our hero, for all they do. They mean everything to me, and I would be nothing without them. Thank you for being by my side and putting up with all my nonsense.

# Contents

List of Tables and Illustrations      11

Introduction      13

1. Autism, the Concept      21

2. The Autism Spectrum      55

3. Etiology of Autism      101

4. Autism through the Stages of Life      129

5. Living and Autism      154

6. Strategies for Daily Life      171

Coda      196

Glossary      200

Further Reading      203

# List of tables and illustrations

## A) Tables

**Table 1.** Comparison of the main defining characteristics
of autism with Asperger's syndrome.                                     62
© Maria J. Portella

**Table 2.** Brief description of the main neuropsychological
symptoms described in different neurological, psychiatric
and neurodevelopmental disorders.                                    96-97
© Maria J. Portella

**Table 3.** Main brain changes and their impact
on behavior in different stages of life.                            112-113
© Maria J. Portella

**Table 4.** Example of a table to identify emotions.                   174
© Maria J. Portella

**Table 5.** Example of a planning matrix to progressively
change restricted activities or behaviors.                             191
© Maria J. Portella

## B) Illustrations

**Illustration 1.** Normal population distribution curves.              52
© Maria J. Portella

**Illustration 2.** Population distribution according
to IQ score.                                                           76
© Maria J. Portella

**Illustration 3**. Representation of the cumulative effect
of emotion dysregulation in autism, in which different everyday
situations increase emotionally dysregulated behaviors until
reaching total meltdown or shutdown.                                    85
© 2018, Chan, KTM: *Rewarding the Autistic through Understanding
the Neural Cognitive, Emotional, Motor binding Circuitry in the
Developmental Brain*. Creative Commons Attribution License.

**Illustration 4**. Diagram of the different neurodevelopmental
processes in relation to embryonic age and after birth.          107
© Maria J. Portella

**Illustration 5.** Stages of embryonic development in relation
to the brain regions that emerge from the neural tube and
approximate age of the embryo.                                          110
[Adapted by Maria J. Portella.]
© 2016, Correll, B. Brain Formation. Available at:
*https://ib.bioninja.com.au/options/option-a-neurobiology-and/a2-the-human-brain/brain-formation.html*

# Introduction

About a decade ago, the National Institutes of Health (NIH) in the United States contacted a group of non-profit and private partners to provide $28 million for a research project to investigate biological markers in autism. The aim was to determine objective biomarkers of autism so that diagnosis would not be based on a behavioral assessment. James McPartland and his colleagues at Yale University developed a detailed project to produce a set of biological and psychological measures to be used as biomarkers and which could serve as indicators for long-term evolution in clinical studies and in drug development.

This fact was an indication of two different aspects: on the one hand, the growing interest in autism over the last decade, whether for social, cultural, biological or scientific reasons; and on the other, the lack of objectivity in diagnosing autism, a condition that, as of today, has no clear biological basis and is based on the clinical eye, that is to say, subjectivity, of who must determine whether a person is autistic or not. And this is a problem, especially for professionals looking to find valid interventions for autism.

Since 2015, knowledge about autism has advanced in many respects, but not enough to have this set of biomarkers on the social and communicative function of autism spectrum disorders, the name under which autism is grouped in the primary psychiatric diagnostic manuals. So how is it possible that, in the second decade of this millennium, the scientific account of autism remains so entrenched in the realm of subjectivity, as is also the case with other diagnostic categories in psychiatry? How can a neurodevelopmental diagnosis be so present and visible, while at the same time so heterogeneous and mysterious? It can be considered unfortunate that autism is detected and identified in such a surprisingly subjective way, or at least in a non-biological or non-scientific way. However, what if the diagnosis and detection of autism moved on a more objective, firmer terrain? How would the findings end up being transferred into the daily lives of autistic people and their families? What would be at stake in trying to make autism a fully biological condition? All these questions cannot be answered solely from the perspective of scientific research, psychology and medicine, as other aspects are involved having to do with the model of intervention and, indirectly, the model of society desired —or imposed— from the centers of power. Therefore, it is necessary to explore what kind of response can be given from medical sociology, anthropology and, why not, from politics (understood as a decision-making process in human groups). That is, in the midst of this tangle of biological certainties and diagnostic ambiguity, other vectors appear that interact and put a strain on some of the more complex aspects and most important issues in these disciplines. Tensions exist between autism and neuroscience, between biological markers and complex conditions, between objective measures and subjective narrations, etc. In short, between the body and life.

All these issues seem to be at a critical point these days, following nearly eighty years of clinical and scientific research. We are at a time when many things are being questioned, when people have a lot of information at their disposal —though not always verified— and people emerge who are experts in everything and nothing. Autism is no exception. Although it was long believed that autism was first described in 1943 by Leo Kanner, an Austro-American psychiatrist, it was Grunya Sukhareva who characterized it almost two decades earlier than the Austrian child psychiatrist based in Baltimore, Maryland. In 1924, a twelve-year-old boy, who was different from his peers in many ways, was taken to a Moscow clinic for evaluation. He showed almost no interest in other people and preferred the company of adults to that of children his own age. He never played with toys: he had learned to read at the age of five and spent the day reading as much as he could. Slender and stooped, the boy moved slowly and uncomfortably. He also suffered from anxiety and frequent stomachaches. Grunya Sukhareva, a young doctor at the clinic, looked him over with a sharp eye and pointed out that he was "highly intelligent" and liked to take part in philosophical discussions. As a diagnosis, she described him as having "an introverted nature, with an autistic proclivity in himself." Interestingly, the description in the clinical picture made by Sukhareva is very similar to the description of traditional autism spectrum disorder. Her original article in a German magazine appeared in 1925, almost two decades before the case reports by Asperger and Kanner. However, Sukhareva's pioneering work was overlooked, probably because of Soviet isolation during the inter-war era and also, perhaps, due to the fact she was a woman.

Around the same time as Leo Kanner, Hans Asperger, another Austrian doctor, observed and described a very similar syndrome at his clinic in Vienna. Although Asperger looked more closely at the strengths and talents of his young patients, the clinical picture he described closely resembled Kanner's. This similarity was not known until Lorna Wing, in 1981, redefined and reintroduced Asperger's syndrome, even though it emerged as an independent diagnosis from autism and was associated with a high-functioning (intellectual) variant of autism. In this era, the influence of American psychoanalysis (which reached its height in the late 1960s) still persisted, and it defended that the origin of the syndrome lay in a poor mother-child relationship. At the time, there was still much debate about the extent to which autism was a "neurological" condition. One of the effects of this assumption was to act as a driver for the autistic community to organize, in the broadest sense, thanks to which networks of people were created who wanted to be part of the world of biological research on autism. Since then, and as a sign of the times we live in, this whole conception of autism has been reviewed, discussed and researched as never before, and with a strong presence by associations of autistic people and their families. Nevertheless, a broad consensus has not been reached among the countless researchers and professionals working worldwide on autism. Nor has this consensus been reached on a more local level, such as in socio-health care or in the educational or occupational programs around us.

When someone with certain knowledge is asked what autism is, their answer is usually that it is a neurodevelopmental disorder with deficits in three core features (also called the autism triad): social interaction, communication and repetitive behavior. You can also say that it is hereditary, and that in a group of 60 to 80 school-age children one can have it, and there is a higher incidence in boys than in girls. However, certain inaccuracies can be found in this description, which could explain why the hoped-for progress is not being made, especially considering the significant economic and personal investment mentioned at the beginning. The first is to only focus on three observable features and not go any further. Interestingly, in the fifth version of the *Diagnostic and Statistical Manual of Mental Disorders* (DSM-5), social communication and interaction have been combined as a single diagnostic criterion, and a single category of autism has been created that includes autism, Asperger's syndrome and pervasive developmental disorder not otherwise specified (PDD-NOS). Another shortcoming is not to have included the characteristics that are typical of females. And last but not least, it once again focuses on autism as a childhood disorder, thereby forgetting the characteristics typical of autistic adults. Even so, the description given at the beginning of this paragraph is the most common internationally and, as such, many diagnoses and therapeutic interventions are based on this concept. Fortunately, more and more evidence and literature are gradually reversing this view of autism.

Understanding what happens to a person whose condition is on the autism spectrum means understanding what happens in their brain, from genes to behavior, but not just that. In other words, in order to understand autism, it must be kept in mind that these people think and act differently, they tend to alter the usual ways of perceiving anything, from politics to the social and personal environment, and even the impact that scientific discoveries can have on their identity and daily life. So much so, that understanding autism also means reflecting on how we use the term to refer to it, whether as a label, as a characteristic, or as a part of someone's identity. For this reason, throughout the text the terms *autistic person* and *person with autism* will be used interchangeably. This is because, far from there being a clear consensus in the group in regard to the condition of autism, it is up to each individual to decide what to call themself or what they want to be called, always respectfully and with dignity.

In short, it is a question of thinking about the relationship between neuroscience and autism, about how researchers who are dedicated to this study, still without biological certainty, reflect on and interpret their results about a being that is constantly changing. This implies having to understand what it means at the intellectual, methodological and emotional level in order to comprehend something as varied, idiosyncratic and heterogeneous as the autism spectrum and fit it into the biological, statistical and material limitations of neuroscience. In trying to explain this relationship, two opposing scenarios can be given: either science is successful and autism becomes a universally discrete, definable and demonstrable category (let's say, "natural") that has only been waiting for knowledge to make it visible; or, with the knowledge acquired —and with the knowledge that continues to be acquired— autism ends up becoming something more "social" (as opposed to "natural"). Sociologists, anthropologists and even philosophers will surely bet on this second scenario, while "hard" scientists might defend the first. Or maybe not. Possibly, it is not a question of establishing a dichotomy but of finding the links between the two scenarios. Or is it that neuroscience (and other knowledge) cannot end up explaining the endless complexity of human social life? Or is it possible that the fact of being social beings who interact will bring forth more elaborate conceptions that require a higher use of brain resources and help us to understand autism and many other things from a non-binary perspective? (The —detestable— dichotomy of knowledge between sciences and letters remains an example.)

Allow me, before we enter the world of autism, to make a brief note. The reader will find that words appear in bold throughout the book. These terms have been considered relevant and are therefore defined in the "Glossary" to facilitate their understanding.

This quick immersion in the still murky waters of autism will lead us to discover how far scientific and social knowledge about this condition has come in the last decade; to find the crux of the matter; and to sketch out some strategies for daily functioning, that is, with autistic people and for autistic people, throughout their entire life.

# Chapter 1
# Autism, the Concept

In his book *Tracing Autism*, the sociologist Des Fitzgerald (2017) asked a group of neuroscientists working on autism what exactly it was for them. From all the answers, it can be established that, in principle, it is a clinical phenomenon reasonably well described and understood. Everyone agreed that it is a disorder within the spectrum of neurodevelopmental disorders with some characteristic impairments in three core features (as already mentioned, the autism triad) of social interaction, communication and repetitive behavior (this is how it is reflected in the *American Psychiatric Association* (APA) manuals in 2000 and, with the exception of communication, also in the manuals in 2013).

Nevertheless, if you look at and consult everything published on autism, you will see that this definition, which has already been detailed in the introduction, does not work well in all cases, nor does it serve to make autism more observable beyond the clinical eye of the professional who must diagnose it. Changes are constantly being made in diagnostic manuals, nuances when establishing neurobiological mechanisms, suggestions are made by expert committees to provide social and health responses, changeable percentages of incidence and prevalence are published, etc. The aspect that leads to the most discussion and lack of agreement about autism is that it is based on this triad, as it does not cover all aspects of the condition. Nor is the specific genetic etiology, which will be described later, useful as it still remains unknown despite all the advances that have taken place. Navigating through all this, divergences concur among schools of thought that discuss whether autism should be characterized as a condition, as a disorder, or, in some circles, as a disease.

What distinguishes these three terms from each other is the relative emphasis that is intended to be made with regard to functional change, structural change, the presence of signs and symptoms and, perhaps to a lesser extent, the seriousness you want to transmit. In the style section of the *American*

*Medical Association* (see *AMA Style Insider*), the following definitions are given based on *The Compact Oxford English Dictionary* (2nd edition); the *Merriam-Webster's Collegiate Dictionary* (11th edition); and the *Dorland's Illustrated Medical Dictionary*:

- *Condition* simply indicates a state of health; a condition that confers pathology could be classified rather as disease or disorder, so this can be used instead of disease or disorder when a neutral term is desired.

- *Disorder* denotes a condition characterized by functional deterioration without structural changes, and although certain disorders or categories of disorders may be accompanied by specific signs and symptoms, their presence is not necessary for a condition to be called a disorder. Like condition, disorder is sometimes used as a neutral term instead of disease.

- *Disease*, on the other hand, indicates a condition characterized by functional deterioration, structural changes, and the presence of specific signs and symptoms. In addition, *Dorland* specifies that the deterioration of functioning associated with the disease may constitute any deviation or disruption of normal function or structure, and also states that the etiology, pathology, or prognosis may be unclear and unknown.

According to these definitions, the three terms would be quite equivalent, although it is true that, in common language, the term *condition* is not associated so much with disease or pathology, whereas *disorder* is. Precisely for this reason, many people prefer to talk about *autism spectrum condition* (ASC) rather than *autism spectrum disorder* (ASD). As according to the AMA style book both terms have this more neutral connotation, when speaking of the more medical concept the term *disorder* will be kept, while in the rest of the chapters it will not be used and, in the case of wanting to speak of the diagnostic category, the term *autism* or ASC will be preferred. In any case, the central theme of this book is autism and autistic people and, as such, we will not enter more deeply into this discussion.

Autism is usually diagnosed in infancy or early adolescence, but it is a lifelong condition that can show an oscillating course. It is inheritable, some neurogenetic components are known, it is diagnosed more in boys and men than in girls and women, and it is very heterogeneous (that is, on the one hand, we can have an autistic person with good functioning and a seemingly typical life, while, on the other, there are individuals who may need constant help throughout their lives). The diagnosis of autism in adults was not often made in the past century, and it is still difficult to find professionals who are able to establish the diagnosis, due to this widespread and misleading conception about it. Even so, in the last two decades there has been an increase in cases of autism worldwide. It is remarkable how, slowly but steadily since the 1990s, the diagnosis of autism has become very visible and present. In 1976, autism had an estimated prevalence of four to five cases per ten thousand children under the age of fifteen (Wing et al., 1976). In 2014, the U.S. Centers for Disease Control and Prevention (CDC) showed a prevalence of one in sixty-eight North American boys and girls aged eight (and one in forty-two boys). What has caused this increase? Some argue that it has been environmental factors such as pollution, but more widespread scientific opinion holds that the increase in the number of diagnoses is instead due to a combination of detection and recognition of autistic symptoms and the "diagnostic substitution" of other classic categories such as "mental retardation" (Frith, 2003). Again, we find that, in the attempt to explain this "autistic pandemic," new scenarios open up to also investigate the increase in awareness and concern about autism from the cultural, social and scientific point of view. And even more important, attention needs to be paid to everything that *has not* been made visible, even though autism has occupied many aspects of the public sphere in recent years.

## The medical concept

Currently, autism is considered a disorder that includes others having certain common denominators, as can be deduced from the DSM-5 diagnostic criteria, which is what is used in our setting. To meet these diagnostic criteria for ASD that appear in the first heading, a child must have persistent difficulties (referred to in the DSM as deficits) in each of three areas of social communication and interaction plus at least two of four types of restricted, repetitive behaviors (in which it is necessary to highlight the inclusion of hypo and hyperreactivity in sensory input or unusual interest in sensory aspects of the environment, which has led to an improvement in recognition of a wider and more "comprehensive" range of other symptoms or other characteristics associated with them, such as anxiety).

In order to include all forms of autism, each of the above points includes the two extremes that were discussed previously. Moreover, it is necessary to specify what level of severity the person shows at the present time, which should be based on social communication impairments and restricted, repetitive patterns of behavior. Again, it is necessary for the severity to be specified under this second heading.

The other headings focus on the fact that symptoms must be present in the early developmental period, although it is noted that they may not become fully manifest until social demands exceed limited capacities, or may be masked by learned strategies in later life —the inclusion of this last note has facilitated, as will be seen below, the diagnosis of autism in females; symptoms must cause clinically significant impairment in social, occupational, or other important areas of current functioning; and these disturbances should not be better explained by intellectual disability (intellectual developmental disorder) or global developmental delay. Intellectual disability and autism spectrum disorder often occur simultaneously; for comorbid diagnoses, that is, simultaneous diagnoses of autism spectrum disorder and intellectual disability, social communication should be below that expected for the general developmental level.

In order to narrow down diagnoses made prior to the appearance of DSM-5, a note was added explaining that people with a well-established DSM-IV diagnosis of autistic disorder, Asperger's disorder, or pervasive developmental disorder not otherwise specified should be given the diagnosis of ASD. Individuals who have marked deficits in social communication, but whose symptoms do not otherwise meet criteria for ASD, should be evaluated for social (pragmatic) communication disorder.

As has been mentioned after some of the criteria, the severity level must be specified in order to make the diagnosis with DSM-5. Three different levels are established for both the symptoms of social communication and for restricted, repetitive behaviors: Level 3 implies that the person "requires very substantial support"; Level 2, that they "require substantial support"; and Level 1, that they "require support." In short, Level 3 implies minimal social communication, with marked daily interference from repetitive/restricted behaviors due to inflexibility and difficulty in changing the focus of attention; at Level 2 there is a marked deficit in social communication and frequent interference from restricted/repetitive behaviors; Level 1 responds to altered social communication that does not require support *in situ*, and the repetitive/restricted behaviors involve significant interference in at least one context. Also taken into account are subclinical symptoms that do not involve significant impairments (such as excessive or highly unusual interests that do not interfere in daily life).

Finally, DSM-5 criteria require specifying whether the ASD is with or without accompanying intellectual impairment, with or without accompanying language impairment, if it is associated with a known medical or genetic condition or environmental factor (these aspects will be discussed in detail later), whether it is associated with another neurodevelopmental, mental or behavioral disorder, and if it is accompanied by catatonia.

At this point, it is worth mentioning the article by researchers Manouilenko and Bejerot of the Göran Hospital in Stockholm (2015), in which they highlight the great similarity between the clinical picture described by Sukhareva in 1925 and the DSM-5 description of autism spectrum disorder described directly above. Although Sukhareva initially referred to the clinical picture she had observed in six boys over a two-year period at the Psychoneurological Department for Children in Moscow as schizoid personality disorder in children or schizoid psychopathy —following the classification systems at that time— she later replaced the term "schizoid psychopathy" with "autistic (or pathological avoidant) psychopathy." On her list she described an autistic attitude, expressed as a tendency toward solitude and avoidance of other people or the company of other children from early childhood; strange and impulsive behavior, which she referred to as "clownish" or "comical" behavior. She also observed that some spoke non-stop or asked the people around them absurd questions. Their emotional life seemed flat, although they often seemed strange. At the cognitive level, the child psychiatrist described a tendency toward abstraction and schematization, which did not improve with the introduction of specific concepts, and which impeded thought processes. In non-verbal communication there was a lack of facial expressivity and expressive movements, the presence of mannerisms (exaggerated or repetitive gestures or expressions), a decrease in postural tone, and a lack of modulation in speech or peculiar speech. Also added were superfluous and synkinetic movements (involuntary movements associated with voluntary movements), the voice usually sounded nasal, hoarse or sharp and often had a lack of modulation.

Regarding interpersonal relationships, Sukhareva observed that these children stayed apart from peers, avoided shared games, and preferred fantastic stories and fairy tales. They had difficulty adapting to other children and were often ridiculed and scorned by their peers. In regard to restricted interests and repetitive behaviors, she described it as a tendency to automatism, that is, sticking with any task begun, showing great inflexibility, and having difficulties in adapting to changes and anything new. In turn, they showed behaviors similar to tics, making a lot of faces, saying neologisms (invented words); they asked repetitive questions, spoke in stereotypical ways, with quick or restricted speech. The emphasis on the similarity of the situations she described as a tendency toward obsessive-compulsive behaviors, to "wasting" a lot of time preparing activities, and to having difficulty in to stop doing a task. The need to follow rules and principles made them seem pedantic and led them to have emotional explosions when faced with changes, that is, getting agitated if interrupted, with the overriding need to start all over again after the interruption. Sukhareva also described an exclusive dedication to their interests, as if they were "stuck," and often they maintained them for a long time, which was combined with a tendency toward rationalization and rumination, sometimes bordering on absurdity. The sensory question was observed in the fact that most of the six boys were musically gifted, had a better perception of tone and, at the same time, showed greater sensitivity to noise and the need to search for spaces that were calmer. They also had greater olfactory sensitivity. Referring to the similarity with the latest DSM-5 criteria, Sukhareva noted that the onset of autistic psychopathy should happen in early childhood, there was an inability to attend normal school because of the strange behavior, and the intellectual level should be normal or above the population average.

In contrast, in other diagnostic manuals or systems, such as the tenth version of the International Classification of Diseases (ICD-10) from the World Health Organization, autism was included until relatively recently under the heading of pervasive developmental disorders (with code F84 in the ICD-10 version). These are a group of disorders characterized by qualitative anomalies in reciprocal social interactions and in communication patterns, and by a restricted, stereotyped, and repetitive repertoire of interests and activities. These qualitative anomalies were a general characteristic of the individual's functioning in all situations. If there was an associated medical condition or mental retardation (unfortunately, this old concept is still used for intellectual disability), the ICD-10 proposed adding codes. In May 2018, the latest version (ICD-11) was published, which also condenses autism, Asperger's syndrome, and pervasive developmental disorder not otherwise specified in a single diagnosis of ASD. This change reflects certain criteria very similar to the DSM-5, but there are some differences between the two classification systems. The ICD-11 proposed detailed guidelines to distinguish between autism with, and without, intellectual disability. By contrast, the DSM-5 simply recognizes that autism and intellectual disability can occur.

Both DSM-5 and ICD-11 assume the existence of childhood disintegrative disorder, a regressive condition that appears at the end of early childhood within the autism spectrum, despite its distinct characteristics. The DSM-5 does not include regression as a criterion for the diagnosis of autism, while ICD-11 lists "loss of previously acquired skills" as a characteristic on which professionals can base their diagnosis.

Unlike DSM-5, ICD-11 does not stipulate that a person must have a certain number or combination of characteristics to reach the autism threshold. Instead, it lists different pathognomonic characteristics and allows the clinician to decide whether or not a person meets the criteria. On the other hand, there is a change in ICD-11 in respect to symbolic play, which is among the criteria for autism in ICD-10. Given that the way children play varies from culture to culture, the ICD-11 puts less emphasis on the type of play and focuses more on whether children follow or impose strict rules while playing, a behavior that can appear in any culture. Insisting on rules and imposing them on others could be a sign of inflexible thinking, which is common among people with autism. The DSM-5 also moves away from symbolic play but includes some criteria based on play, such as difficulties in sharing imaginative games or making friends and a lack of interest in their peers. Therefore, the two manuals try to adopt criteria that can be translated between cultures. Just as the DSM-5 does, the ICD-11 stresses the importance of assessing unusual sensory sensitivities, which are common in people with autism. It also alerts clinicians to the fact that some people on the spectrum try to mask or camouflage their autistic characteristics, a criterion that is making diagnosis in girls and adults a bit easier, as will be seen later.

The changes introduced in the ICD-11 in comparison to previous versions did not cause the same controversy as happened with the appearance of the DSM-5. At that time, some researchers, professionals, and affected people feared that people classified as Asperger's syndrome or autism spectrum not otherwise specified would lose access to services and end up becoming invisible. It seems that these concerns have diminished and there have been no reactions in this regard.

We could continue to list many other classification systems that depend on public administrations or are more private initiatives, but all would lead us to the same conclusion, which is that it is still not clear whether autism is, or is not, a single condition that encompasses different clinical pictures or syndromes. One of the most surprising aspects for the uninitiated who enters the field of autism is to realize all that is missing from really knowing about it. Perhaps even more significant, however, is the extent and proliferation of explanatory gaps among the characteristics that are indeed supposedly known. Of the few aspects that in principle we could know, such as what causes autism, how it affects cognition, or even how it is "noticed" in someone who is diagnosed, we continue to be unable to advance in how other aspects connect or interact with what is already known on any other level. It is possible for a person to exhibit similar idiosyncrasies in communication and interaction, but in the end they are not necessarily indicators of a cognitive or neuropsychological problem. Any one of us can show some very restricted interest or laugh in a more exaggerated way or not make friends very easily. So, it seems that autism also entails a certain gradation, as has been seen in the different classification examples, and, at the same time, also requires a greater accumulation of these idiosyncrasies, which all manifest themselves almost simultaneously, to be able to make the diagnosis.

Ultimately, to put it simply, what all this is reflecting is the heterogeneity of autism that experts so regret, and which is evident in many different aspects. Autism is heterogeneous in regard to symptomatology: it has already been seen in the diagnostic triad (until it is finally replaced) of social interaction, communication and repetitive behavior that the symptomatology can appear to varying degrees in diagnosed people. There is also heterogeneity, as noted above, in the functioning of a diagnosed person in what some call the "neurotypical" or "normotypical" world (for example, the world of people with "normal" development). In the words of Patricia Howlin, currently one of the best experts on autism, many people diagnosed with ASD live perfectly independent and ordinary-looking lives; others, however, will never talk and will require permanent attention. And finally, there is heterogeneity in its causes; for example, autism is considered highly inheritable but, so far, very specific mutations have only been found for a minority of cases, as will be seen later.

## The legal concept

With the Optional Protocol to the Convention on the Rights of Persons with Disabilities, adopted in December 2006 at United Nations headquarters in New York, the first comprehensive human rights instrument of the twenty-first century was established. This represented a paradigm shift in the approach to policies on disability, moving beyond the health care viewpoint to address another that was based on human rights with an explicit social development dimension. Subsequently, United Nations General Assembly Resolution 67/82 expressly recognized the need to promote and protect the human rights of all people with autism spectrum disorders, and to ensure equal opportunities for them to reach their ideal development potential. Resolution 67/139 designated April 2 as World Autism Awareness Day, which has been celebrated since 2008.

The Charter of Rights for People with Autism, which was adopted in the form of a declaration by the European Parliament on May 9, 1998, sets out the rights that must be upheld by the legislation of each country in the European Union (EU). Disability policies continue to be the responsibility of the Member States in the European Union, who locally implement educational, health and social regulations as well as provisions for autistic people. The formulation of these policies throughout Europe has been changing over the years in favor of autistic people, and will surely continue to change, depending on successive governments, with the not inconsiderable risk of experiencing a setback in the achievements of recent years.

Today, the rights of autistic people are generally respected, but there is still room for improvement. Far from having regulations in common, policies differ enormously between countries such as the United Kingdom, France, Poland and Spain, to cite just a few examples (Roleska et al., 2018). However, there are also differences among regions in the different countries, like in the United Kingdom, where the Autism Act was implemented at different times. This law on autism, which establishes that there must be a government strategy to improve services for autistic adults and serves to provide legal guidance to city councils on how to implement actions, was implemented first in Wales and England (2009), and then later in Northern Ireland (2011). This law sets a review for every five years or so to update the legal strategy and guidance, which provides the possibility to make changes that adapt to needs as they arise. Nevertheless, getting aid is very complicated and, in fact, the results of a 2018 report from the National Autistic Society noted that up to 71% of autistic adults in England did not receive the aid or support conceded to them by the National Health System.

In the case of the Spanish state, in 2011 laws were adopted that adapted to current regulations in the International Convention on the Rights of Persons with Disabilities, but it was not until the end of 2015 that the Spanish Strategy on Autism Spectrum Disorders was approved. The objectives were aimed toward promoting respect for independent living, autonomy, full participation and inclusion, equality, accessibility and non-discrimination. Unfortunately, the Strategy was not implemented, as it depended on an Action Plan that, as of mid-2021, is still pending development. As in the case of the United Kingdom, there are differences between the autonomous regions on which the Health and Social Affairs portfolios depend, despite the fact that they end up being governed by the same laws. As such, divergences are most likely to be found during implementation and in the offer of assistive services. In this sense, the French model managed from the *Secrétariat D'État Chargé des Personnes Handicapées* would be comparable, since the national strategy on autism is applied in all regions under the same general guidelines.

What can be read between the lines in these regulations, laws and decrees is that the public administration is very prepared to accompany autism in the early stages of life, but not so much in adults who, without legal and assistance coverage, see how they cannot make their own decisions and exercise their rights (in Spain, a big opportunity was lost with passage of Law 15/2015 on voluntary jurisdiction, as it did not regulate the full exercise of rights and equal legal capacity of people with Autism Spectrum Disorder). And this happens whether or not they have a recognized degree of disability, because they have never been included in any care plan. So much so, that some pieces of legislation are partially or totally ignored in most EU countries, and there is no equal opportunity for autistic adults as they do not have access to specialized services nor to the labor market. In the United Kingdom charities play an essential role, much like associations and foundations in other places, and end up covering the needs that are ignored by the public administration.

Within this legal perspective on autism, it is necessary to pause to take a look at disability as a legal-administrative concept. The document adopted by the convention mentioned at the beginning recognizes that disability is not the result of sensory, physical, mental or intellectual "dysfunction," but is the result of the interaction of the limitations this entails with the barriers that society imposes for full and effective participation on an equal basis with the rest of the people. What this definition wants to reverse is the fact that people with disabilities, like other historically discriminated groups, have been denied, and continue to be denied in most parts of the world, social, legal and moral membership in society on equal terms. However, some autistic people refuse to wear the label of disability out of shame and due to the stigma attached to it, despite these attempts.

Linked to the concept of disability and with reference to the above-mentioned article 12 of the Convention, the question of civil incapacitation arises. By establishing the need to transform decision-substitution models, such as civil incapacitation, into decision-support models for effective recognition of persons with disabilities on equal terms, a contradiction emerges with the classifications that many states impose to receive aid according to the degree of disability. The debate on the need to eliminate incapacitation, as proposed by the Convention's "paradigm shift," starts specifically with the legal doctrine, without a dominant consensus as debate is divided on this issue. This is surely a reflection of the dichotomous reactions that incapacitation causes in society: some perceive it as a civil death, while others consider it a tool for protection.

Be that as it may, in the current legislation of some EU states, disability is a continuum that usually goes from 0 to 100%. A person is placed on this continuum, which is determined by an assessment given by the corresponding administrative bodies. Recognition of the degree of disability can be sought by all people who show diagnosed and documented congenital or acquired diseases that cause deficiencies expected to be permanent in nature and involving a restriction or absence of the capacity to carry out daily activities, in the way or within the margin that is considered normal. Recognition of the degree of disability is, ultimately, an administrative document that legally certifies degree of disability and facilitates access to different rights, services, programs and assistance aimed at compensating for social disadvantages arising from disability or for the social barriers that limit full and effective participation in society. According to the assessment, there are categorizations in each country from which possible aid comes and which constitute reference patterns for allocation of disability percentages. These percentages are determined in accordance with the criteria and classes specified in each regulation for each one of the deficiencies. The International Classification of Functioning, Disability and Health (ICF) from the WHO is the international standard to describe and measure health and disability. This was formally adopted by the 191 Member States of the WHO at the Fifty-fourth World Health Assembly on May 22, 2001. This classification establishes different classes of health and moderate disability (corresponding to percentages of 0 to 50%) and classes of permanent and severe disability (with percentages of about 50 to 74% and 75 to 100%, respectively). Variations in the classification system between the different states are minimal, but compensation plans do indeed differ greatly among developed countries (in the case of the United States, most of these plans are with private coverage).

Legal status as a person with a disability is accredited when it reaches a percentage equal to or greater than what is established by each state (in Spain it is 33%, while in France or Germany it is 50%). Degree of disability introduces the figure of assistance or compensation for disadvantages, in keeping with the convention, but does not break with the dominant binomial of guardianship/curatorship. Currently, in the case of autism, the degree of disability is linked to the level of severity of the symptoms listed in the diagnostic criteria (explained earlier with the DSM-5). In some countries, such as Germany, the autism diagnosis is automatically given a degree of disability of 30% and is revised upwards based on the difficulties observed. In Spain, however, a case of autism with intellectual disability or delayed language development having Level 3 (requires very substantial support) will probably be given a disability above 50%, while an autism compatible with Level 1 Asperger's syndrome will be given a disability below the established limit and will therefore be left out when it comes to receiving much of the aid.

A reflection on the terminology around this topic leads us to the need to rethink the concept of disability, perhaps adopting the term "functional diversity," as the Independent Living movements have already done, which is associated with more inclusive concepts. Within the concept of disability, the possible typology that connects deficiency and functionality is often pointed out. This establishes physical, sensory, communicative and speech disability, intellectual disability, and the disability arising from a mental disorder.

Different foundations and associations around the world are calling for recognition of **social** or **functional disability** as a new typology that better reflects autistic characteristics. In cases of Level 1 and 2 autisms (requiring support or substantial support), the typology applied is that of intellectual disability or disability arising from mental disorder when often they are neither the one or the other, and this is linked to the resistance to being classified as disability in legal terms. Due to difficulties in verbal and non-verbal communication and social relationships, restricted interests, inflexibility of thought and behavior, among others, the typology of disability would be more of the social or psychosocial type (that is, of adaptation to the daily environment). The lack of legal recognition of this typology implies discrimination of a group with specific characteristics that are, in the end, invisible difficulties, due to lack of knowledge, and which can affect all stages of life. Even so, it remains a controversial concept.

A final but no less important aspect of the legal concept of autism is the relationship with the law. There is considerable evidence that people with disabilities are involved in crimes at higher rates than those without disabilities. People on the autism spectrum are generally very obedient from a very young age and have difficulty picking up on ulterior motives, so along with potential cognitive or intellectual disabilities, they end up being easy targets for abuse and victimization. Unfortunately, most of these cases are never properly prosecuted, so the perpetrators continue to victimize other vulnerable people. The situation is more complicated when the perpetrator of the crime is the autistic person.

Due to their nature, autistic people may show varying degrees of understanding of the criminal justice system or of the situation that has brought them before the law. It is usually very difficult to obtain accurate accounts of the crimes and for victims to be adequately represented and their rights safeguarded. For this reason, it would be good to bear in mind some of the behaviors that autistic people can show in an encounter with officials from the judicial system, whether they are victims or perpetrators of the crime. Above all, care should be taken not to misinterpret some of these actions as being deliberate, disrespectful or hostile. Some examples would be:

- having trouble communicating the facts because their way of describing, for example, abuse, may not be what is expected, which means their account is often questioned;
- not understanding their rights and not knowing what is expected of them;
- failing to respond to verbal instructions given to them;
- running or moving away when justice officials approach;
- being unable to communicate with words, repeating only what is said to them, or just saying yes or no to any question they are asked;
- avoiding eye contact while, at the same time, not respecting personal space;
- acting petulant or stubborn;
- being too sensitive to flashing lights, sirens, crowds;

- being cognitively blocked due to feeling anxious or agitated, so they react with fight or flight responses, shouting, hand-shaking or self-injurious behavior;
- can appear to be under the influence of narcotic or intoxicating substances and suffering from seizures;
- looking at a single object and asking questions repetitively;
- speaking in a monotonous voice with unusual pronunciations, confusing personal pronouns or subject pronouns when speaking (saying "can I stop?" instead of, "can it stop?"), or speaking in an inappropriate volume;
- being honest to the point of severity or rudeness;
- not being able to communicate the extent of the trauma because of a lack of understanding of healthy sexuality or appropriate boundaries;
- and finally, not knowing about the criminal justice system and the expectations and potential consequences that help in the prosecution.

Thus, it is essential to provide information about autism to jurors, prosecutors and defense lawyers, as this can reduce the number of questions and relieve concerns about the competence of the person involved. Unfortunately, incorrect perceptions about autistic people often call into question their credibility as witnesses. But don't forget that autistic people have a very good memory and pay a lot of attention to detail, which makes them reliable witnesses; however, they can be easily confused in adversarial proceedings if they feel pressured or the environment does not seem understanding and patient. As people may be intimidated by aspects of the criminal justice system, by repeated interrogations or the presence of the perpetrator of the crime, it is essential to familiarize them with the environment and prepare them for testimony.

Legal changes are not always enough, given that the prevailing mental framework is a society built from "normality" and by means of a capacitism that seems to confer moral and legal superiority on "us" to the detriment of those labeled as "others," those who are different, the disabled. This paternalistic perspective does not allow full understanding of autism, and for this reason other views are necessary to understand its scope.

## The social concept

Beyond the medical and legal conceptualization, one of the questions that arises is whether everything can really be included in autism. It is not an exaggeration to say that autism has currently become fashionable, and the number of diagnoses, associations and its media presence have grown.

There are different possible answers to this question: that in fact autism is not necessarily one thing, in the way one sometimes imagines —this is where we can find sociological arguments to broaden this view. Another answer is that autism is a clinical sign —observable manifestation— within a broader psychiatric conception, in which diagnoses are defined according to their probabilistic relationship with other signs on different levels (which would be the mechanics of the proposal on Research Domain Criteria, RDoC, from the National Institute of Mental Health in the United States, for example). And a third argument would be related to the conception of autism as a single "diagnostic category" or as a list of symptoms, and that any other approach would be mere speculation. But we have already seen that the last two answers have led us to where we are now, to this categorical medical concept that, nevertheless, has some unclear limits.

As for the first response, there have been different attempts throughout the brief history, and often in parallel with the "advances" in more empirical medicine and psychology, to establish the sociological factors of autism. As the different disorders that fall under the autism umbrella are characterized by difficulties in social interaction and communication, different studies within the social sciences have been defending the need to reconceptualize autism outside the "intrapersonal" domain and direct it toward the sociocultural area. Most scientists, and also sociologists, have tended to place autism in the domain of psychology and medicine and, as a result, autistic perception has become stigmatized. This has resulted in the exclusion of autistic perspectives when it comes to producing knowledge about the experiences lived by autistic people. The first-person accounts examined in certain studies support the idea that **symbolic interactionism** provides a more nuanced framework for studying how autistic perception influences autistic experience, in contrast to the functionalist-reductionist approach of cognitive psychology or the more biological approach of neuroscience.

From this perspective, autistic differences would be defined by disposition and interaction, socio-culturally speaking, rather than simply as a result of individual cognitive or neuropsychological impairment. The application of more sociological concepts in autistic perception and interaction would have the potential to broaden the knowledge on both the autistic experience and the social construction of legislation. It would be like explaining autism from itself and its relationship to the world. Strange as this may sound, Jessica N. Simpson has written a doctoral thesis on this social concept of autism. As she herself describes, most studies on the self and autism have been based on Baron-Cohen's Theory of Mind (TM) concept and have focused on the difficulty of autistic people to deduce the mood of others (Baron-Cohen, Leslie and Frith, 1981).

From the start, the author disputes the role of TM in explaining or understanding autism. According to her, very little research has attempted to clarify how or what autistic people think about themselves and their relationship within the social world. The consequence is that autism is understood to result in distinctive personal development, and studies have focused on these differences as deficits and dysfunctions. One criticism of this framework, therefore, is that what is considered pathological deviation is the result of larger social forces that describe the parameters of normality.

To what extent can this social conceptualization of autism help to understand it? It is difficult to answer this question, but what is certain is that it could have extraordinary consequences at all levels. First off, it is a radical approach to a much commented but poorly understood concept, as it enters fully into the social debate about autism: questions are posed such as, What does it mean to have a "self"?   or, What does it mean to not have a "self" like the majority of people?, as if wanting to say that some people do not have the necessary components for personality, relationships, equality and, therefore, humanity. Autistic autonomy is guided from the alternative framework of **symbolic interactionism**, and the discussion is transferred from the neuropsychological and cognitive spheres toward the sociocultural sphere. The aim is to demonstrate how, from a sociological perspective, the difference in itself is not sufficient to imply a deficiency, a problem, a pathology. In fact, these differences, according to this view, have resulted in stigmatization of autonomy and of the way autistic interactions are done.

Sociological thinking about identity therefore poses a big challenge in the diagnosis and treatment of autism. In spite of this, the most basic questions about autism and the broader implications they pose are the most intriguing. Sociologists have made and continue to make important contributions to research on autism and they have placed it in broader social contexts, including institutions that help (or do not help) autistic people and the inequalities that can occur in access to treatment.

And here, above all, there is an opportunity to learn more about the interactions between socialization and genetic inheritance. Perhaps as sociologists spend more time seeing how autistic children are taught to navigate the social world, or how teenagers and adults try to have more stable personal relationships, they will find interesting examples showing how socialization, despite disability or difficulties, still determines a large part of who we are.

## The concept of neurodiversity

Within this current that includes more sociological aspects, or at least further removed from the clinic, different associations and writers, among them Steve Silberman, reinterpret and attempt to show how the stereotypes associated with the medical-psychological concept of autism prevent our culture, as a whole, from reaching its full potential. In Silberman's book entitled *NeuroTribes*, the author attempts to convince readers of how the most audacious and avant-garde science and innovation has been shaped by autistic people. And he uses a very interesting concept, that of **neurodiversity**, the idea that neurological and neuropsychological differences such as autism, dyslexia, attention deficit hyperactivity disorder (ADHD), are not errors of nature or products of the modern world but rather the result of natural variations in the human genome. The term *neurodiversity* refers to the variation of the human brain in terms of sociability, learning, attention, mood and other mental functions. It was coined in 1998 by sociologist Judy Singer —who is autistic— and she popularized the concept with journalist Harvey Blume. The idea behind this is that conditions such as autism should not be seen as disabilities, but as perfectly normal neurological and neuropsychological differences between people.

Here, perhaps, you start understanding that this more "comprehensive" conceptualization could change the rules of the game, if it isn't already doing so today. As we begin to better understand how these variations can provide certain skills and abilities, which are usually extraordinary or not very common, it will be necessary to reassess the educational system and establish the basis for a cultural change that recognizes and "celebrates" a wider range of ways to perceive the world. Nevertheless, we still do not understand what neurodiversity is because we remain stuck in very Cartesian thinking, rigid to a certain extent, that does not let us understand the series of unique options and profiles that exist within the human species.

One way to represent this change is that in normal distribution (in the statistical sense) of human characteristics within the population, the different neuro-diverse conditions would be placed on the **bell curve** (i.e. **Gaussian distribution**) as variations of the human species (see illustration), and not as separate groups in the way that health, education and social systems have, in essence, been proposing for decades.

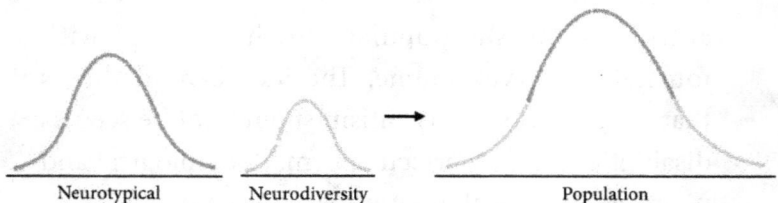

Neurotypical          Neurodiversity                    Population

**Illustration 1.** Normal curves of population distribution. On the left, neurodiversity is represented as a different group from neurotypical, according to models of segregation, and on the right, the inclusive and integrative proposal, in which the difference lies in the frequency of occurrence of neurodiversity in the general population.

This view proposes a review of the medical model of disability that describes the person with a disability as a type of deficit; the ultimate goal of the doctor is to eliminate or reduce this deficit and make the person "as normal as possible." In particular, neurodiversity is rooted in the social model of disability, which considers it rather as a civil rights issue. The social model rejects the notion that an individual must be "neurotypical" to enjoy the full range of human experiences, arguing that an impairment should not constitute a barrier to inclusion or access.

Disability, therefore, stems largely from society's failure to adapt to diverse needs. This does not mean that all deficiencies are caused by external factors, nor that we should not try to address them through medical means if these are beneficial for the person. Rather, it means that, while a person experiences an impairment, society must work to support and accommodate them.

This impairment in autistic people is often seen, for example, in how they are disproportionately affected by external sensory environments, which can overwhelm them to the point of experiencing a **meltdown** or **shutdown**. Anxiety is also a factor that should be taken into consideration, as will be seen later. However, because most neurotypical people do not easily recognize these difficulties (called *invisible disabilities*), the behaviors of autistic people are often misunderstood and interpreted as "difficult behaviors." Advocates of neurodiversity consider these to be problems of accessibility to various supports. Recently, you can hear more talk about boys and girls with special educational needs and of how, often, they are much more likely to be permanently excluded from regular schools. At the same time, however, it is not so common to hear comments about the fact that this is perhaps a problem that has to do with accessibility and that the right of these children to an education, or of adults to the world of work and leisure, might be being violated. At least, this is what is being criticized from the position of neurodiversity, and it certainly contributes a different perspective on awareness about autism.

# Chapter 2
# The Autism Spectrum

It was not until the late 1970s that autism was reconceptualized as a developmental disorder and, recently, it is also being referred to as a neurological-based (Damasio and Maurer, 1978) and genetically-based disorder. However, it is still considered that autism can be represented as a continuum (a continuous line) in which nonverbal autism with intellectual disability would be at one extreme and high-capacity autism with intact verbal communication would be at the opposite end. That is, autism would range from high functioning to severe disability. Those described as highly functional would be defined as being verbal, having higher than average intelligence, and having few social and communicative disorders requiring accommodation. In contrast, severe or low-functioning autism would be characterized by serious learning problems due to intellectual disability, lack of communication due to language delay, and many social deficits. Thus, depending on complexity and severity, people with multiple social, communicative and physical impairments would normally be considered at the lower end of the spectrum, while those with high functioning would be at the upper end. Some autism experts have argued that this language and this conceptualization reinforce the idea that autism is bimodal. Terms such as *high functioning* and *low functioning* represent a picture of autism that denies the strengths that may be present in low functioning autistic people, while highlighting the challenges facing those labeled as high functioning. These terms are considered offensive and are believed to overshadow the nature of autism.

At the same time, this dichotomous or bimodal conception is based on a single axis that would simultaneously include the autism triad. This means that, if a person shows stereotypy but has an interest in other people —despite not having success in personal relationships— it would be hard for them to be diagnosed with autism. One of the most-repeated cliches by certain professionals who lack sufficient knowledge is that if the person is able to look in the eyes of their interlocutor, they cannot be described as autistic. The fact of wanting to apply the triad in such a limited way within this single continuum caused autism to be under-diagnosed for many years, since only those cases that corresponded perfectly to their, let's say, classical definition (the one popularized by Leo Kanner) were detected.

It is in this context where considering autism as a spectrum comes in, a spectrum with different dimensions that can be more or less branched off from what is considered normal or less frequent (for a detailed explanation on the concept of normality see *Mundos Invisibles* by the same author). At the same time, it also responds to another confrontation between two opposing positions: either autism is a discrete biological entity, the causes of which will one day be discovered with the right tools (medical concept), or autism is a temporary and contingent set of symptoms, whose classification probably navigates free from any biological substrate, specifically the brain (social concept).

What is contributed by describing autism as a non-linear spectrum? The meaning of spectrum is the representation of the decomposition of a compound wave into simple wavelengths of particular frequency. It is usually applied to the electromagnetic spectrum, which is the decomposition of electromagnetic radiation, to the solar spectrum, which refers to the decomposition of solar radiation, or also to the acoustic spectrum, which is the set of sound waves of well-defined frequencies that make up a sound by superimposing. Visible light is a small part of the electromagnetic spectrum, with wavelengths that cover a range from between 400 to 800 nm. In short, a spectrum is made up of different waves with different overlapping wavelengths. The key, then, lies in the decomposition of different waves (which we could assimilate with signs and symptoms) with different wavelengths (a more or less pronounced impact on the life of the person and their environment) that can overlap or combine.

Perhaps the spectrum of visible light is a model that can help to better understand this explanatory approach. Laurence Arnold, a former member of the National Autistic Society of the United Kingdom and an autism expert, described his own autistic experience by focusing attention on the fact that the literature describing autism, the symptoms, and autistic perceptions is often too simplistic, does not represent them and conflicts with the real experiences of autistic people. Therefore, a more nuanced understanding of autism leads to regarding it not as an entity with degrees of severity, but rather as a set of traits that manifest in different degrees for each individual, some of which are not entirely unique to autism. There are those who represent it as a mixing console (or audio mixer), in which behavior, language, emotion, communication, sensitivity, cognition, etc., would be the input channels and each person would have a position at the controls (the faders on the console) that is different from the rest, and which could change over the course of life in the same person.

Defining autism as a spectrum is to conceive that someone who shows differences in some areas of human functioning (which include from language and perception to motor skills, mental functioning, the senses, etc.) may not show differences from the stereotype of a person in other areas. In other words, no longer considering that there are slightly autistic people (with "good functioning") and very autistic people (with "low functioning"), but rather that within the spectrum there are different features or ways of using the brain to process the information around us (both information gathering and response); some of these traits involve many difficulties in everyday life —and are therefore diagnosed— while others may be very useful for the person's daily activity.

Each autistic person has a range of characteristics in the different areas of the spectrum. In areas where there are no autistic traits they can function like neurotypical people, although they may be affected by circumstances in other areas. This shows that no autistic person acts exactly like another, despite having certain factors in common. This conception is explained very well in comic format at www.the-art-of-autism.com, where Rebecca Burgess makes the comparison with a color palette and the different areas of brain functioning. And by using drawings, she offers many enlightening examples: such as, an autistic person can be a very good conversationalist. Nevertheless, places with noise and a lot of people can overload them so that finally they cannot carry on a conversation at that moment; not all autistic people have some type of talent; or, with an autistic person who cannot communicate verbally, this does not necessarily mean they cannot understand what they are being told and need a different way of communicating.

In no way is this a denial of the presence of disability in autism. On the contrary, it is understood that different people need different kinds of support and that aid for mental and physical health are equally important. The intention is to make it clear that disability is not a competence, and that society plays a relevant role when it comes to determining the extent to which difficulties may be more or less disabling to the individual.

## Autism and Asperger's syndrome

One of the issues that continues bringing about heated debate is the difference, if any, between autism and Asperger's syndrome. Lorna

Wing's reintroduction of Asperger's syndrome did not associate it so closely with autism, but rather presented it as a different category. In fact, Asperger's syndrome was added to the DSM-IV in 1994 (in the version prior to the current one) as a separate disorder from autism. The few professionals who worked on it considered Asperger's syndrome to be simply a milder form of autism and used the term "high-functioning autism" to describe these people. Uta Frith, professor at the Institute of Cognitive Neuroscience at University College London and editor of the textbook *Autism and Asperger Syndrome*, described people with Asperger's as "having a touch of autism."

The latest decision to have only one category for autism in the DSM-5 was based on terminological accuracy: the experts who participated considered that all these diagnoses should be merged into a single category of "autism spectrum disorders" and argued that creating a broader spectrum "would help diagnose children with autism more accurately and coherently." And in this context, the debate is once again deafening. If one searches in any source looking for the difference, you will find very specific lists of the signs and symptoms that separate them. In the following table, you can see some of the areas where there would be differences between the two clinical pictures, but they do not have a consensus among researchers nor do they have scientific studies to support them:

| Autism | Asperger's syndrome |
| --- | --- |
| Is a mental condition present since early childhood. Characterized by great difficulty in communicating, having relationships with others, and using abstract language and concepts. | Is a neurodevelopmental condition related to autism. Characterized by peculiarities in social interactions, pedantic language, and preoccupation on very restricted interests. |
| Much more serious clinical signs and symptoms. | Much milder signs and symptoms. |
| They prefer to be isolated from society. | They prefer to be in society and interact with others, no matter how difficult they find this. |
| There is a delay in language development. | There is good language development, although its use is peculiar. |

**Table 1.** Comparison of the main defining characteristics of autism with Asperger's syndrome.

It would seem that the two conditions really can be quite well differentiated, at least on paper. There are other "experts" who even distinguish between Asperger's syndrome and high-functioning autism (even if this differentiation between high and low-functioning in autism creates little sympathy in some sectors). The divergences would lie in the nature of the not-so-restricted or obsessive interests, in the possibility of delay in language development, and in the normal development of motor skills in high-functioning autism.

Nevertheless, even though there are people who use these small differentiations, the fact is that there is no longer a diagnosis of Asperger's in the DSM-5 nor in the ICD-11. The signs and symptoms that were previously part of the diagnosis for Asperger's are now included within the autism spectrum. People who had previously been diagnosed with Asperger's are now diagnosed with autism spectrum disorder.

But many people who were diagnosed with Asperger's before the diagnostic criteria changed in 2013 are still perceived as Asperger's or Aspies —as many of them call themselves— and this is in line with the fact that being an Aspie forms part of their very identity. This fact is undoubtedly related to the stigma that still surrounds diagnoses of autism in many societies around the world. Despite this, the only real "difference" between the two diagnoses is that it can be considered easier for people with Asperger's to "pass" as neurotypical, only showing "mild" signs and symptoms that might resemble those of autism. Later on, we will discuss whether this idea of having it easier is really like this or not.

The evidence used to gather all these conditions under the same umbrella of autism, according to Catherine Lord, one of the members of the working group that reviewed the diagnosis, shows a strong bias from professionals. In a multicenter study that investigated the differences in a diagnosis of Asperger's in twelve centers, which professional had made the diagnosis was the factor that best predicted these differences: what is known as *interviewer bias.* This result is worrisome, as it demonstrates that the phobias and philias of the evaluators were more important than the presence or absence of characteristic symptoms. There was also a social class factor in a number of the centers included in the study. Children of upper-middle-class parents were diagnosed with Asperger's. The same child with the same characteristics, but with less educated parents, would end up being diagnosed with pervasive developmental disorder not otherwise specified. This is not good. Medically and scientifically there was no justification, according to Lord, to have a separation between Asperger's, pervasive developmental disorder not otherwise specified, and autism. She also states that the working group did not in any way attempt to be "provocative," and the benefits of the newly diagnosed criteria are clear. "We're just saying there are more examples organized in a different way, that we think will identify people with ASD and do a better job of not identifying people who don't have ASD."

There is another parallel reason, from recent history, to argue for the "elimination" of Asperger's syndrome as a diagnosed entity, which was developed by the historian Edith Sheffer in her essay "Asperger's Children: The Origins of Autism in Nazi Vienna" (2018). This is a compelling exploration of the history of Hans Asperger. Hans Asperger has long been considered one of the advocates for defense of children with disabilities because of his contribution to autism. However, after an extraordinary search, Edith Sheffer reveals how the Viennese doctor not only participated in the racial policies of the Third Reich in Hitler's Nazi Germany, but also, as the author explains, was an accomplice in the murder of boys and girls. As has been widely documented, the Nazi regime, in addition to killing millions of people throughout Europe, devoted itself to classifying people according to race, religion, behavior or physical conditions in order to treat them or, rather, eliminate them. Nazi psychiatrists focused on children who were different (especially those who had no social skills) and stated that they had no place in the Third Reich. Asperger and his colleagues made an effort to shape some autistic children into productive citizens and, if unsuccessful, sent them to the Am Spiegelrund Children's Hospital in Vienna, where 789 patients were killed under Nazi Germany's system of childhood euthanasia. The appearance of this essay stirred the conscience of many people, and many voices requested that the syndrome not have the Viennese doctor's name. Other options were proposed, such as calling it Sukhareva's syndrome. Even so, and with removal of the diagnostic category from the DSM-5, this change has not flourished beyond certain associations and activist blogs.

The consequences of including Asperger's syndrome within the autism spectrum —and thus eliminating its diagnosis— are not entirely clear, as there are all types of opinions. As the new criteria reduce the number of symptoms within each category while increasing the number needed to make the diagnosis, by effectively limiting the "menu" of options some critical voices note that the only thing that has been achieved is to make the diagnosis more restrictive. Other researchers and professionals argue that any decrease in the number of diagnoses should be very modest, or perhaps that diagnoses could even increase, according to criteria from the DSM-5 or ICD-11. Many experts have confirmed that this revision is in no way intended to leave people out of the spectrum, but rather is about further refining the diagnosis to make it more useful and representative of the data collected over the last twenty years. Ultimately, the members of the commissions, who reviewed and created the versions of the DSM-5 and the ICD-11, did not find enough differences between autism and autism not otherwise specified or Asperger's syndrome, but their advocates were not sufficiently satisfied either, as Brian King states in an opinion article.

Moreover, the uncertainty —as researchers seem to be shaping diagnostics "on the fly"— has not been much to the liking of some members of the passionate community of parents of autistic people, nor for adolescent and adult Aspies themselves. They fear that if they are awarded good functioning and less severity they may lose the —scarce— aid in education, social services, pensions, etc. Many are also concerned that elimination of the Asperger's diagnosis will seriously affect the sense of identity of some individuals in the autistic community, even if it does not result in a reduction in the above-mentioned services. However, we should not forget that the reference point for diagnosis is a broad spectrum with different key aspects that overlap and interact in daily functioning and give rise to unique and characteristic patterns. If this heterogeneity is taken into account and restrictive criteria are avoided, no autistic person should be left without a diagnosis.

## Autism in women

Throughout the book, and especially in this section, the distinction between man/woman, boy/girl is used with the criterion of majority biological sex and not of gender identity to facilitate reading. The author is fully aware of the gender perspective and how it affects neurodiverse people.

Nonetheless, it appears that autism is more common in boys/men than in girls/women, and that professional researchers are beginning to better understand the differences in the way in which each one manifests autism. Although this is promising for future generations, girls/women still have certain problems in getting a diagnosis and finding treatment.

Vanessa is a New York-based writer who discovered when she was already an adult that she was Asperger's. For this reason, in addition to books, she often writes texts on healthline.com in the section on autism. Her article *Why I Fake Being 'Normal' and Other Women with Autism Do, Too* begins as follows:

> When I first learned that I had Asperger's syndrome and was "on the spectrum," as people like to say, I read anything I could get my hands on. I even joined an online "support" group for people with autism. While I recognized some of the traits and issues described in articles, journals, and the support group's community forum, I could never fully see myself in any of it. I couldn't check all the boxes that would wrap up my personality into a neat package with a warning label that read, "Fragile, handle with care." As far as I could tell from what I was reading, I wasn't at all like all the other autistic people in the world. I didn't fit in anywhere. Or so I thought.

Later she goes on to say: "Usually, people don't think I'm on the spectrum at all, mainly because it doesn't always look the way they think it should. Plus, I'm really good at altering my behavior to mimic conventional social norms —even when it feels odd to me or is contrary to what I actually want to do or say. Many autistic people are." And here you can add, above all, women. In this sense, a study published in the journal *Autism* in 2016 found that, on average, autistic women showed more "camouflaging" behaviors than autistic men. Examples of camouflaging include making eye contact during conversation, use of learned phrases or prepared jokes in conversation, imitation of others' social behavior, facial expressions or gestures, and learning and following social scripts. This could be one of the reasons why fewer women are diagnosed with autism or take much longer to be diagnosed.

Rates of the prevalence of autism —that is, the proportion of individuals diagnosed at a given time— suggest that boys are, on average, four times more likely to be autistic than girls. However, this figure may hide the true incidence of autism in girls and women, with some estimates ranging from 7:1 (for example, 7 boys for each girl) to 2:1. A relevant fact is that many times parents with daughters on the spectrum share frustrating stories about the difficulties as well as the impossibility of getting a proper diagnosis for their daughters, while many autistic women did not receive a diagnosis until adulthood.

Nevertheless, is it true that autism is more common in men? One curious fact is that three decades ago there were practically no diagnoses of autism in women, but studies have now lowered the ratio to two boys for each girl. It has been shown in several studies that the fact of being a woman appears to protect the brain from many developmental disabilities, not just autism. There is much evidence coming out that shows girls with autism need more extreme genetic mutations than boys to develop it. However, there is a growing field of research in the last decade that indicates autism presents differently in girls and, as such, is often not recognized, especially in girls with verbal fluency and normal intelligence. Meanwhile, there is also the fact that diagnostic criteria for the autism spectrum is largely based on how it presents in men, and therefore girls can often "fly off the radar" of the criteria or get a wrong diagnosis. Autistic girls/women appear to have less restricted and repetitive behaviors than boys/men, and some of these behaviors may not be recognized as an obsessive interest: for example, collecting dolls can be misinterpreted as a simulation game.

Beyond the possible differences between men and women with autism, there is a very relevant differential aspect, namely that autistic girls/ women are more vulnerable to internalizing symptomatology such as anxiety, depression and eating disorders. As more is learned about autism in women, the importance of early diagnosis becomes apparent, as well as the need for effective support and greater understanding. In fact, researchers in the 2016 study found that constant camouflaging behaviors often imply costs such as exhaustion, increased stress, feeling defeated due to social overload, anxiety, depression, and even a negative impact on development of their own identity.

Some researchers have hypothesized that this gender difference may be related to the X chromosome, while others highlight the role of the level of intrauterine testosterone. It is possible that current diagnostic criteria is slanted toward a male stereotype of autism and is less appropriate for recognizing it in women. It is not surprising, then, that it is often the "least feminine" women —according to majority cultural constructs— who have been diagnosed with autism. In one of the talks at the International Meeting for Autism Research in 2009, researchers Dworzynski and Ronald presented the results of a study investigating the effects of gender on autism spectrum disorders, alluding to differences in symptoms and intelligence in a sample of twins. First, they confirmed previous findings: In the general population, total autistic traits were more evident in boys than in girls, and the IQ was lower in girls diagnosed with autism than in boys. Nevertheless, and this is the interesting point, the fact that girls who were undiagnosed, but with marked autism traits, did not show any disadvantage in IQ could suggest that the likelihood of a diagnosis is affected by the IQ level in girls more than in boys. In other words, autism, and especially the more subtle forms of autism, may be more difficult for experts to recognize in girls/women, mainly with the presence of normal or high intelligence.

A few years later, in 2012, the study by these two researchers, along with cognitive neuroscientist Francesca Happ of King's College London, compared the occurrence of autism traits and formal diagnoses in a sample of more than 15,000 twins. They corroborated their earlier results. That is, if boys and girls had a similar level of these characteristics, girls had to have more behavioral problems or significant intellectual disability, or both, to be diagnosed.

Going back to the question of higher frequency of autism in men than in women, scientists have investigated several explanations over the past two decades about the amount of gender bias in autism. In this process, they have discovered, beyond social and personal factors that can help women mask or compensate for symptoms of autism better than men, biological factors that might prevent autism from developing. The main theory is the "extreme male brain" from Simon Baron-Cohen, which first appeared in the literature in 2002 and is still a subject of study. The idea is that autism is caused by fetal exposure to higher-than-normal levels of male hormones, such as testosterone. This occurrence forms a mind more focused on "systematizing" (understanding and classifying objects and ideas) than on "empathizing" (taking into account social interactions and other people's perspectives). In other words, autistic minds would be more powerful in areas where the male brain, on average, tends to have strengths and less powerful in areas where women, broadly speaking, are the superior sex. (On an individual scale, needless to say, these averages say nothing about the ability or capacity of a specific man or woman, nor do they necessarily reflect an immutable biological determinism with no role from the culture.) Some scientists, among them Baron-Cohen, think that extreme male brain theory could explain sex/gender differences. In contrast, a second idea arises when looking at the most powerful brain areas of women. If having female hormones and a female brain structure increases the capacity to read other people's emotions and makes social concerns more prominent, a larger number of genetic or environmental impacts may be needed to alter this capacity to a sufficient level to be able to "detect" autism. This idea is known as the "female protective effect" theory. If either, or both, of these theories is correct, there will always be more boys than girls on the spectrum. And as Baron-Cohen says, "I imagine that once we're very good at recognizing autism in females, there will still be a male bias. It just won't be as marked as four to one. It might be more like two to one."

A final point worth mentioning is the relationship between anorexia and autism. In the mid-2000s, researchers led by psychiatrist Janet Treasure of King's College London began exploring the idea that anorexia could be a possible manifestation of autism in women, another factor that would make them less likely to be identified as autistic. According to Kate

Tchanturia, a colleague of Treasure and researcher on eating disorders, there are striking similarities in the cognitive profiles of both conditions. People with autism as well as those who have anorexia tend to be rigid, with very detail-oriented attention, and they are distressed by changes. Some research exists suggesting this connection between anorexia and autism. In another study by Baron-Cohen and his colleagues in 2013, a group of 1,675 adolescent girls (66 of whom had anorexia) was evaluated and they measured to what extent they showed different autistic traits. The research found that the women with anorexia showed higher levels of these characteristics than the typical women did. This relationship is not especially strange, as many people with autism find certain food tastes and textures aversive —as an example of hyper- or hyposensitivity— and often end up with very restricted diets. This does not mean that most women with anorexia also have autism. A meta-analysis done by Tchanturia and her team in 2015 put the figure at around 23%, a rate of autism far higher than what is seen in the general population. What all this suggests is that some of the spectrum's "lost (undiagnosed) girls" might have been diagnosed with an eating disorder.

There is still a long way to go; social and cultural constructs related to gender and behavior do not help much, as they make it difficult to recognize signs of autism in girls and women.

## Autism and intellectual capability

Intelligence, as defined in "Mainstream Science on Intelligence," is a very general mental capability that, among other things, involves the ability to reason, plan, solve problems, think abstractly, comprehend complex ideas, learn quickly and learn from experience. It is not merely book learning, a narrow academic skill, or test-taking smarts. Rather, it reflects a broader and deeper capability for comprehending our surroundings. Individuals differ from each other in these domains and, at the same time, intellectual capability can vary in the same individual depending on the circumstances and how these domains are evaluated.

The quantitative assessment of intelligence is done via the IQ obtained by administering tests that examine the different cognitive domains, including tests with verbal content (related to the use of language in both comprehension and production) and performance tests (related to spatial and abstract processing). The test scores obtained are then transformed into an IQ scale and the individual score is compared against a standard (Gaussian distribution or bell curve), taking 100 as an average and a standard deviation of 15. Thus, scores between 85 and 115 are considered normal (68.2% of the population), whereas an IQ greater than 130 is considered very bright and below 70 is referred to as mental retardation or intellectual disability.

Similarly, disability has varying degrees ranging from mild (IQ between 70 and 55), moderate (54-40), severe (39-25), and profound (below 25). As you can see in the following illustration, only a very small percentage of the population has scores below 55 or above 145.

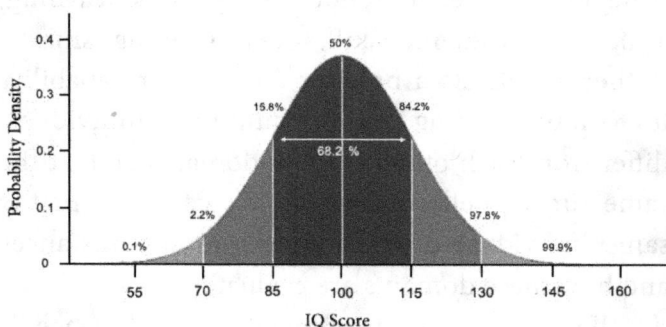

**Illustration 2.** Population distribution according to IQ score. Percentages indicate the amount of the population that is below each score.

For a long time, autism was considered to be closely associated with intellectual disability (formerly known as "mental retardation") and a characteristic intellectual profile predominated, with better performance in manipulation testing and poor performance in verbal skills, apart from a distinctive pattern of "peaks" and "valleys" in the set of tests included in assessment of intelligence. One fact that was widely accepted is that up to 75% of people with autism had an intellectual disability.

However, many of these views had not been substantiated and were also based on a conceptualization of autism that does not correspond to the current one; the historical data on prevalence and incidence that determined these percentages of intellectual disability cannot be applied to boys and girls (nor to adults) who are currently diagnosed with autism. Thus, in a 2011 epidemiological study, Charman et al. found that in a representative sample of boys and girls with autism about 55% had an IQ below 70 (for example, intellectual disability), and only one in five had a severe disability; approximately 16% had a below-average IQ (between 71 and 84) and the rest a normal IQ, and only 2.7% had above-average intelligence. Another fact confirmed was that more girls than boys had intellectual disability, but this result would end up being questioned because of the insufficient sample of girls included in the study and for the reasons noted above.

Early signs and presentation of autism differ if the condition is accompanied by intellectual disability. In these cases, the characteristic signs of autism are associated with those that are typical of disability, such as generalized developmental delay in psychomotricity, communication, curiosity, sphincter control and, in general, in the capability for functional adaptation. We can say, in these cases, that the early signs of autism appear sooner or, in other words, they can be detected earlier. In those with cognitive ability that falls in the normal range, the first signs identified have a "more autistic" quality and are not so related to cognitive ability. In general, some autistic people with preserved intellectual capability and good development of expressive language are identified through problems with sociability and pragmatic communication, difficulties in adapting to rules, in understanding a new environment without their adult references, and difficulties later on in joining games like their peers, despite the fact that, in other cases, these problems have already been seen at the start of primary education.

For this reason, it is highly relevant to evaluate intellectual capability since, without being defining, it is a good predictor of how the rest of the difficulties and characteristics of the autistic person will manifest themselves. It is necessary to re-emphasize the fact that autism can occur at any point on the IQ continuum, and having a high or low intellectual level does not necessarily make the individual more or less autistic, although it can indeed have implications on what each person's life will be like within the spectrum.

## The other characteristics of autism

There are diverse voices that express disagreement on classification systems for autism, as current criteria continue to leave out many other defining aspects. Autism does not generally arrive alone. Usually, it is linked to other diseases, disorders, conditions, etc. Unfortunately, this is not taken into account when making a diagnosis and, often, the presence of these characteristics masks the core symptoms of autism, whether because they overlap or because when faced with a lack of knowledge labels are given that are easier to handle. When the autism spectrum has been discussed, other aspects have been introduced beyond communication and restricted behaviors (it is worth remembering that language stopped being one of the core symptoms in the new versions of the DSM and the ICD). It is also about broadening the view in secondary colors and giving them the importance they deserve to better characterize autism and facilitate more valid and comprehensive coping strategies. To sum up, the following illustration, adapted from the review published by Dr. Chan from Hong Kong, shows the wide range that goes beyond the autism triad, giving an idea of the difficulties and complications that can be involved from the point of view of diagnosis, treatment and prognosis of autism.

It could be considered that restriction of the medical concept of autism is what has led to these other aspects not being included in the definition, in the sense that neuroscientific and sociological advances have not been incorporated. But it could also be, when the voice of autistic people has been listened to, that professionals have begun to realize the main difficulties are not found exclusively in the triad but rather affect virtually all facets of human life. When these aspects are not taken into consideration and are not specifically addressed, the likelihood increases of difficulties becoming symptoms and the mental health of autistic people being greatly affected.

## Emotion dysregulation

Emotion regulation is the individual's capability to respond to the demands of an experience with the internal and external world by means of a set of emotions in order to be socially tolerable and flexible enough to allow spontaneous reactions. It is also the capability to delay or convert —eliminate— spontaneous reactions depending on the setting and context. It is the set of processes responsible for controlling, evaluating and modifying emotional reactions. Within regulation there is also emotional self-regulation, which includes both regulation of one's own feelings and the regulation of other people's feelings as well. It is made up of three factors that are intertwined: cognitive, related to problem-solving strategies and flexibility; emotional processing, to identify one's own emotional signals and those of others; and neurobiological factors, which include the brain structures involved in both executive functions and emotional processing.

In contrast, emotion dysregulation is the term used in mental health referring to emotional responses that are not well modulated and not found within the range of what is socially acceptable. Possible manifestations of emotion dysregulation include extreme weeping, angry outbursts, destructive behavior or throwing objects, aggression toward oneself or others, and threats to commit suicide. Emotion dysregulation can cause behavioral problems and interfere with a person's interactions and social relationships at home, at school, or at work. It may be present in people with attention deficit disorder or hyperactivity, bipolar disorder, borderline personality disorder, etc., and also in those on the autism spectrum.

Even so, this characteristic does not appear among the diagnostic criteria in autism and, more importantly, as a therapeutic target for interventions. And it's not for lack of evidence. In a very interesting 2013 study, Andrea Samson and her colleagues examined the relationship between emotion dysregulation and the basic characteristics of autism spectrum disorder. They developed an emotion dysregulation index that included most of the behavioral impairments described by different experts in child and adolescent evaluation. Their results showed that, compared with the control subjects, autistic children and adolescents had more emotion dysregulation and significantly greater symptom severity on all scales. Furthermore, emotion dysregulation was related to all the basic characteristics of autism, but the strongest association was with repetitive behaviors. This happened at the same time the DSM-5 was published, but even so, including emotion dysregulation as a diagnostic criterion or as a target for treatment was not considered.

In the book *Mundos Invisibles*, the author already placed special emphasis on emotion dysregulation. It is known that the autism triad is intrinsically related to the use of emotion regulation strategies such that, for example, a lack of understanding of interpersonal relationships, restricted interests, and rigidity of thought do not allow the use of cognitive reevaluation. In other words, autistic people do not have the capability to find alternative explanations that make them feel better about what is happening in their environment and, therefore, end up emotionally overloaded. Another example is the minimal use made of behaviors aimed at an objective or the search for social support when they are in more uncontrolled situations; rather, they use behaviors to compensate for the anxiety the situation creates in them, which are often unexpected and not very effective (such as repetitive behaviors, sounds or screams to keep from feeling things, or self-aggression).

Despite not yet being recognized as a core symptom of autism, diverse studies have already described how the three factors (cognitive, emotional and neurobiological) allow for a better understanding of the entire repertoire of autistic characteristics. Not only that, but the inclusion of emotion dysregulation conceptualizes autism as a much more general condition, thus minimizing the supposed heterogeneity that was explained above. In other words, growing recognition of the impact of severe emotional impairments on autism is being determined by initial empirical findings suggesting that inappropriate emotional responses —for example, emotion dysregulation— can contribute to impaired functioning and, consequently, affect the long-term prognosis. And this puts all "types" and "degrees" of autism on an equal footing. Nevertheless, this is not to say that the severity of symptoms in each of the fundamental characteristics of autism, including impairments in social and communicative functioning, repetitive behaviors, and sensory abnormalities, are not related to high emotion dysregulation. Different studies from the research group of Dr. Laudan Jahromi at Columbia University have shown the connection between poorer social skills (such as lack of theory of mind or inability to have perspective) and greater emotion dysregulation, as well as evidence of the link between emotion dysregulation and low prosocial commitment in people with autism.

The consequences of not taking into account emotion dysregulation as a diagnostic criterion or core characteristic of autism can become the central problem for suffering and discomfort due to the appearance of other psychopathological symptoms and psychiatric disorders. In fact, some voices have already pointed out that if the autistic person could live in an "ideal" environment where they did not have to face changing or incomprehensible situations, were not judged because of their strange behaviors, or could feel good about themself, they would surely not experience so many episodes of emotion dysregulation. Given that this environment does not exist, and it does not seem feasible to create it within the societal model we have, it is essential that attention be paid to one of the characteristics that has the most impact on the lives of these people, either by recognizing it to facilitate contexts such as autism-friendly environments, or by learning how to control it so that it does not go further and end up being a life problem such as, for example, the development of serious psychiatric disorders. Some examples of the effects of emotion dysregulation on the lives of people, both children and adults, are difficulties in sleeping, feelings of resentment that persist over time, strong arguments about issues that are not very important, impairment in social functioning (making friends or keeping them), at work or school (it may be hard to focus on tasks), abuse of substances such as alcohol or other drugs, increased self-harming, alterations in food intake (whether eating restrictively or overeating), tendency to be defiant (especially children and adolescents), etc.

Emotion dysregulation in autism often has a cumulative effect; people enter spirals of incomprehension, either because of conflicts or social situations, due to changes in the environment or because of sensory overload that makes them feel even more uneasy, as nothing they put into practice helps them feel better. Recent studies have found an interaction between social motivation —wrongly thought to always be low in autism— and emotion dysregulation: it interferes with children's ability to take advantage of their social motivation, as they have few social skills, even when they have relatively high social motivation. Jahromi's group has expressed this through a scale in which emotion dysregulation increases until the emotional explosion appears, which manifests itself as a meltdown or shutdown.

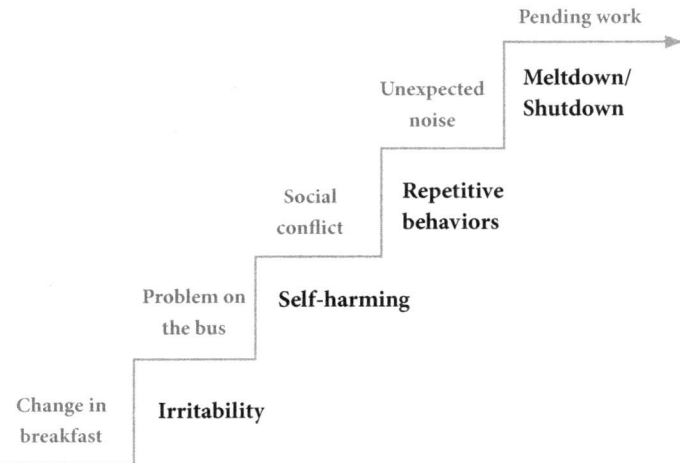

**Illustration 3.** Representation of the cumulative effect of emotion dysregulation in autism, in which different everyday situations (in gray) increase emotionally dysregulated behaviors (in black) until reaching total meltdown or shutdown.

Another characteristic related to emotional regulation that deserves a separate comment is alexithymia, which is the difficulty in understanding, processing and describing emotions. This is manifested in 85% of autistic people. It has been proposed that, in the first months of life, when ordered mental states associated with concepts or words are not yet possessed, the most basic emotions are lived through the body. New, more complex emotions are later incorporated, such as desire, surprise and anger, which are also manifested through somatic sensations. During language acquisition, these organic sensations are associated with words and concepts that give them meaning in a coherent and adaptive set, with a common code to identify them in other people, until one becomes a social and reflective being. It appears that, in autism, and in other neurodevelopmental conditions, the brain structure does not allow this orderly formation. For quite some time, this characteristic led to the misconception that autistic people did not have emotions, when in reality they refer to them through bodily sensations but without the sensations being able to access the mental states that the rest of humans share through language.

At the extreme opposite end of emotion dysregulation is another type of emotional response, which is a flat affect. Despite not being very common, some autistic people do not show the usual signs of emotions such as smiling, wrinkling their nose or raising their voice, and they seem indifferent or as if they have no reaction. Sometimes this flat affect makes it difficult to diagnose autism because it resembles a simple schizophrenia. But it can also make it difficult to diagnose other symptoms like depression in autistic people, because they may not show the usual external signs. This is why it is important for professionals and caregivers to check if there are changes in sleep, hunger and general mood.

## Anxiety

Although anxiety is not considered a core feature of autism either, 40% of young people with autism and, according to a recent study by Dr. Nimmo-Smith, more than 20% of adults with autism have an anxiety disorder (also obsessive-compulsive disorder, OCD) or at least clinically elevated levels of anxiety. Some studies have indicated that up to 86% of people have more than one clinically relevant episode of anxiety in their lives. Diagnosis and treatment of anxiety is crucial as it greatly affects basic aspects, such as repetitive behaviors and social problems but also other elements, such as mood and motor activity.

Autistic people have the same concerns and fears as everyone else. But they may also worry or feel stressed about things that are less worrying for neurotypical people. Some examples include the following:

- small alterations in their routines and new sensations that they feel in their body;
- unknown or unpredictable social situations;
- situations where it is difficult to know what others think or feel;
- their own thoughts and feelings, especially unknown or unpleasant physical symptoms related to worrying.

When autistic people are worried or anxious, their way of showing their anxiety resembles characteristics that are typical of autism, but perhaps more intensely: **stimming**, obsessive and ritual behavior, increases and resistance to changes in their routine is more pronounced. That is, anxiety can take unusual forms in people with autism, turning uncertainty or incomprehension into a constant concern. Also, because they usually have trouble recognizing their own anxious thoughts and feelings, they do not always look like anxious behaviors. Instead, they end up showing a wide range of behaviors and reactions that are unexpected, such as an increase in defiant behaviors. These behaviors include: a greater emphasis on routine and situations with the same conditions; the appearance of sleep problems; emotional collapses or explosions; a tendency to avoid or stay clear of social situations; and increased obsessions and rituals, such as aligning, rotating or chopping objects. Body rocking or flapping can also be more apparent, especially in children and adolescents, as well as self-injury by hitting their head, insistent scratching with nails or other objects, or biting their hands or arms.

As a result, because anxiety symptoms are present in most people with autism, they find these highly distressing and a source of many of the functional problems in everyday life. Dr. Isabel Paula of the University of Barcelona is one of the experts who has most underscored the tandem stress/anxiety and autism. Her book *La ansiedad en el autismo: comprenderla y tratarla* (*Anxiety in Autism: Understanding and treating it*) combines the data provided by scientific research with a qualitative approach to how people with autism experience daily, ongoing stress, with increased vulnerability to anxiety. It is not entirely understood why anxiety is still not considered a core symptom of autism.

In recent work by Dr. Paula herself, they have investigated whether the lack of tolerance for uncertainty shown by autistic people could intervene in anxious responses. The conclusion they reach could not be more interesting, which is that probably the alterations in predictive skills in autism can explain the relationship between greater intolerance to uncertainty and some peculiarities inherent in autism, such as behavioral patterns, restrictive and stereotypical interests and activities, and peculiarities in processing sensory information. Thus, and in line with other researchers, it could be thought that the triggers for anxiety in autism would be the autistic characteristics themselves, resulting in an anxiety that is qualitatively different in how it emerges and manifests itself.

Described among the triggers for anxiety in autism are social anxiety, perfectionism, communication difficulties, rigid or inflexible thinking, and unforeseen events (that is, something new or surprising). It has been proposed that the way in which nerve connections are established in the autistic brain (these processes will be explained later), that is, with ample branching but poor specialization, results in certain situations ending up triggering anxious behaviors. The grouped and specialized nerve fibers of neurotypical brains allow a great range of situations to be automated and internalized, so we can respond to them without paying too much attention and, thus, quite effectively and without anxiety in a constantly-changing environment. By contrast, people with autism, apparently having many more but less specialized nerve fibers, experience every situation as if it were new, and thus again need all their resources to deal with them, to develop a response that is more or less appropriate, which greatly increases **arousal** and stress levels, and for this reason anxious behaviors appear.

Anxiety in autism thus has some prototypical manifestations that do not always resemble the most characteristic of anxiety, which include the cascade of physiological changes (sweating, trembling, etc.), cognitive (concern for physiological changes interpreted as a heart attack, "and what if ...”), emotional (fear, panic, etc.) and behavioral (avoidance, flight, etc.) typical of the anxious response. The evidence points to much more exaggerated fight or flight responses in autism, more marked hypervigilance, anger and, as noted at the beginning, increased “autistic” behaviors.

Several hypotheses have been proposed: the first is the social error hypothesis, which defends that maladjustments in the social behavior of people with autism, which arise from impairments affecting the processes involved in social cognition, contribute to exacerbating anxiety in autism. The second is the **allostatic load** hypothesis, in which anxiety is the response to chronic stress, to wear and tear or exhaustion that causes hyperactivation of certain structures in the limbic system, and to the low specialization of the autistic brain. They are not contrary hypotheses. Rather they complement each other, although we still have few studies that can confirm their validity. In this sense, a 2018 study by Schulz and Stevenson found that sensory hypersensitivity, along with emotional overload, led to increased levels of anxiety, which indirectly increased repetitive behaviors and stereotypy in people with autism.

## Sleep disturbances

People on the spectrum, both children and adults, tend to have trouble sleeping, especially in the form of insomnia: it takes them longer than typical people to fall asleep and many wake up frequently during the night. It is estimated that this affects from 40% to 80% of people with autism. In children, insomnia is ten times more frequent compared with neurotypical children, and often this rate continues during adolescence and adulthood. In addition, they may also have sleep apnea, a condition that causes them to stop breathing several times during the night. This can worsen certain aspects of their condition, such as repetitive behaviors, which in turn can make sleeping even more difficult. Given this disruptive feedback loop, sleep problems become one of the most urgent concerns for autistic people and their family or others who live with them. Despite this, it has been one of the least studied aspects of autism.

The origin of sleep disturbances is still unknown. That is, it is not known whether this forms part of the set of impairments in autism or is rather a consequence of them. Many of the conditions that accompany the autism spectrum, such as gastrointestinal, immunological, dermatological or hyperactivity problems, anxiety and depression, by themselves are known to alter sleep. There is some literature suggesting that people with autism are more likely than neurotypical people to have mutations in genes that govern the sleep-wake cycle or are related to insomnia. Some studies even suggest that a high percentage of people on the spectrum have mutations that affect melatonin levels, one of the hormones that controls sleep. Be that as it may, it is one of the problems that really should be taken into account, as lack of restful sleep complicates and exacerbates the most maladaptive and problematic behaviors of autistic people. Improving sleep does not mean solving all the negative aspects of autism, as noted by Angela Maxwell-Horn, a pediatrician at Vanderbilt University in Nashville, but it indeed can improve quality of life. In fact, a study has shown that children with autism who manage to sleep regularly are able to learn more, are less irritable, and have fewer behavioral problems. In another study with autistic adults, they investigated two characteristics that could be relevant because they block achieving an optimal sleep-wake circadian rhythm: greater visual hyperreactivity in daylight and more difficulties in interpersonal relationships, both due to a lack of social skills and lack of sleep-wake patterns adapted to the environment.

## Irritability and aggression

Irritability and aggression are symptoms that can complicate adaptation at home and in other settings, and can manifest themselves as physical or verbal attacks, tantrums, and self-injurious behaviors. Rage is not unusual in people on the autism spectrum. It can appear suddenly, apparently from nowhere, and then disappear with the same speed. Triggers include stress, sensory overload, perception of being ignored, and changes to routine. The intensity, frequency and severity of the behaviors can be different for each person. Behaviors may also vary depending on the environment, such as at home or at school, and also over time.

One study reported that up to 20% of children with autism showed symptoms of irritability and aggression, including attacks, severe tantrums, and deliberate self-harming behavior. Because of the large disruption these can cause, professionals have tried various medications to reduce irritability, such as antipsychotics, antidepressants, antihypertensive agents and others. The results are not as positive as could be expected, and currently more focus is being put on non-aggressive containment and psychotherapeutic techniques to control impulsiveness.

Some people consider that irritability is rather a consequence of the other disturbances in autism and, therefore, what is contributing to it can be determined, such as non-restorative sleep, constipation, various pains or changes in the environment. In this context, psychotherapy and coping strategies are understood to be more effective.

On the other hand, in a recent study of networks, which is an analytical technique that allows the strength of the relationships between different factors to be established, Hirota and colleagues described how symptoms of irritability that were strongly related to each other were associated with more aggressive behaviors (for example, showing aggression through temper tantrums was more frequent in individuals who presented various symptoms of irritability). They thus concluded that early identification of irritability in this population could avoid aggressive behaviors with more serious consequences. In addition, a depressed mood and oppositional behaviors were identified as being bridge symptoms. Interestingly, network structures do not differ between individuals with intellectual disabilities and those without. These findings indicate that addressing bridge symptoms through integrated care that combines different treatment modalities could lighten the complicated network of symptoms and, as such, reduce symptoms of irritability and aggression in people with autism.

## Cognitive dysfunction

Executive dysfunction, dyspraxia, dyslalia, dyslexia, dyscalculia, inattention, prosopagnosia, etc. All these terms are examples of the different cognitive disorders that autistic people may have to a greater or lesser degree, regardless of their intellectual capability. Nor are they properly included in diagnostic criteria. However, they are increasingly recognized by both clinical and scientific professionals, thanks in part to the role of neuropsychology. Each autistic person may have all, some, or none of these symptoms, so it is essential to detect them in order to understand many of the behavioral aspects and frustration that suffering from these cognitive difficulties can create. The most widespread explanation, which will be addressed in more detail in later chapters, is poor development of the neural pathways between different brain regions. This implies difficulties in processing multiple information simultaneously, since sequential and conscious, not automatic, processing is done, which slows cognitive performance. The following table briefly explains each of these symptoms:

| | |
|---|---|
| **Executive dysfunction** | Difficulties in successfully selecting and controlling behaviors that facilitate achieving chosen or completely new objectives; it is not possible to make simultaneous use of different executive functions such as planning, attention, inhibition, cognitive flexibility, etc. |
| **Dyspraxia** | Problems in motor coordination that affect daily activities. |
| **Dyslalia** | Permanent or transient difficulty in the correct pronunciation of certain phonemes. |
| **Dyslexia** | Difficulty in identifying, understanding and reproducing written symbols. Reading is not overall but rather syllable by syllable or sound by sound. It is also manifested by omission, substitution or reversal of letters. |
| **Dyscalculia** | Difficulties in learning mathematics and would be equivalent to dyslexia. |

→

| | |
|---|---|
| **Inattention** | Difficulties in selecting certain external stimuli at the time of perception, being unable to devote the cognitive resources to their production. |
| **Prosopagnosia** | Selective alteration in the perception of faces, which prevents the recognition of one's own features or those of others. |

**Table 2.** Brief description of the main neuropsychological symptoms described in different neurological, psychiatric and neurodevelopmental disorders.

The cognitive dysfunction that has received the most attention from researchers is dysexecutive syndrome or executive dysfunction. As early as the 1990s, Ozonoff, Pennington and Rogers developed the theory of executive dysfunction to explain the restricted and stereotyped patterns in autism. This theory is currently useful in explaining other characteristics of autism thanks to the neuroscientific advances that took place in what was known as the Decade of the Brain. Lack of cognitive flexibility (often referred to as rigidity), planning or temporal organization would not only explain restricted interests and repetitive behaviors, but would also be involved in the difficulty of adapting to changes, as more than one instruction could not be followed simultaneously, in sensory saturation facing a high presence of stimuli, or in the difficulty of perceiving the changing social clues in any interpersonal relationship.

Typically, researchers refer to executive function as the "CEO" of the brain, or as the orchestra conductor, because it is responsible for setting objectives, planning and managing to do anything. Executive function is, as we have already seen, a set of processes and not so much a general skill. It is important to recognize the complexity and involvement of our executive functioning in absolutely everything we do during the day in order to realize the number of problems that can result if these processes are not working properly, as happens in autistic people.

Executive dysfunction in autism, in addition to explaining many of its characteristics, leads to difficulties in stringing together actions aimed at achieving long-term objectives; problems in organizing materials and establishing schedules (two essential aspects in the educational stage as well as when working); problems in controlling emotions or impulses (due to lack of inhibitory control); and difficulties in analyzing or processing information, especially if it happens through different sensory channels and in parallel.

Some examples illustrating executive dysfunction in people on the autism spectrum are:

- they may perceive small details but have difficulty seeing how they all fit into a larger picture, unless there is external support to help them structure its parts;
- they may have trouble maintaining a thought, and this can lead to problems in following simple directions having more than two steps.

For example, they may forget instructions such as "go to the warehouse and bring back the delivery notes" when they arrive at the place they have been told to go to;

- they have trouble planning, organizing or sequencing thoughts; also paying attention. This can lead to problems completing daily tasks, such as getting dressed, getting ready or cooking;

- they show difficulties facing any type of change. This can lead to the appearance of "stubborn" behavior, because the person becomes stuck on a small detail or routine and will not move forward unless the routine is fulfilled. For example, an individual may have problems with an unexpected change in the school routine, such as replacing gym class with a school assembly, or another person may have difficulty finishing a meal if the food is not placed in a particular way;

- they may have difficulty working on a team or with others on a project, either because they may find it difficult to change their own ideas (or receive feedback) or because they cannot integrate the ideas of others;

- they may not be able to react to an accident or incidental event, and they may even make the situation worse by not knowing how to solve the problem in a planned, strategic way.

- they have difficulty flexibly paying attention

to different aspects at the same and may have
little resistance to distraction and interference;
- they can show little ability to manage time;
- finally, and in relation to emotion dysregulation,
they may have difficulty controlling impulses
or regulating behavior when they are upset or
frustrated.

As with other characteristics that have been
described, until very recently professionals working
on autism did not consider cognitive dysfunction
—unless it was specific, such as dyslexia or
prosopagnosia— when considering interventions
and treatments. Surely the fact that it is not seen as
a symptom on the spectrum leads to the fact that
this list of problems and difficulties is still being
ignored. Fortunately, advances in neuroscience,
and in particular neuropsychology, are changing
the landscape of interventions, and there are
already programs and therapies that have executive
dysfunction —the cognitive function that most
alters the daily functioning of the people suffering
from it— as a therapeutic target.

# Chapter 3
# Etiology of Autism

Possibly the most surprising change of all has been the shift from seeing autism as a disorder involving social, behavioral and communicative difficulties to a view that considers it a developmental condition that involves, besides the difficulties mentioned above, perceptual and cognitive impairments that most likely originate from some form of organic dysfunction in the brain which happens during formation of the individual's nervous system. The day when biomedical research offers us the biological truth about autism is still far away, but it is becoming increasingly evident that this thing we call *autism* is the result of multi-level interactions between genes, environments and behaviors, and it is highly unlikely that each of these levels has a unique biological identity.

In general terms, found within the causes of autism —what is called *etiology* in the life sciences— are variations in the genes, in neural pathways, in neurotransmission (the communication between neurons), as well as environmental factors. Although the causes are still not clear in the majority of cases, doing a review helps to better understand the condition as well as its incidence and prevalence. In other words, searching for the causes is currently one of the most effective ways available to understand autism.

## Genetic variations

In a 2010 review of various research studies in both quantitative and molecular genetics, Dr. Jessica Schroeder along with other collaborators (York University in Toronto) showed that autism is polygenic (that is, different genes are involved), with up to 20 chromosomes implicated (of the 23 pairs we have!); specifically, they determined that chromosomes 1, 2, 4, 7, 13, 15 and 16 were the ones that consistently showed a relationship with autism. At the beginning of the millennium, it was already estimated that approximately 70% of the variance in autism was due to genetic factors.

More recently, scientific findings have pointed to new variants that are normally distributed in the population with multiple genes involved, which together can either present *de novo* genetic mutations (not inherited from the parents) or can indeed be inherited, as well as also chromosomal abnormalities. Epigenetics is a discipline that studies how the environment and an individual's history influence expression of the genes and how acquired characters are transmitted from one generation to another; it is the study of reversible changes in gene expression without the nucleotide sequence being altered, and chromatin folds have also been studied in relation to autism, although the results are still inconclusive.

It appears that with autism there are different related mechanisms involving hundreds of genes, with polymorphisms distributed normally in the population that cause additive risk effects. On the other hand, in autism associated with intellectual disability there are genetic mutations and also chromosomal abnormalities involved. Ten percent of autism cases are associated with syndromic causes, of identified monogenic causes, such as fragile X syndrome, phenylketonuria, tuberous sclerosis, Rett syndrome, etc. Five percent are associated with rare chromosomal abnormalities, such as with 15q11-q13 duplication inherited from the mother, trisomy 21, Turner syndrome (45X), 47XYY, 47XXY, etc. Another 5% are associated with variations in the number of copies of parts of the genome, which are repeated more or less times, commonly referred to as copy number variation (CNV), particularly those CNVs that are rare or uncommon in the population: 16p11.2, 7q11.23 duplication, 22q11.2, 15q13.3, etc. Another 5% are associated with penetrant and rare genetic variants in the population (some of the genes associated with brain development are detailed in the next section). The other 75% are, in principle, unknown multifactorial causes, with environmental factors that modulate genetic expression and factors such as paternal age, which could be associated with an increase in genetic mutations. The genetic risk of recurrence, once you have an autistic child, may vary according to the different genetic etiologies involved and be lower in cases where *de novo* genetic variations develop in the affected child.

In a study published in 2019 in the prestigious journal *Nature Medicine*, an international team of scientists —led by researchers from the University of California School of Medicine in San Diego, and with participation from doctors Hervás and Arranz from the Fundación Mutua in Terrassa— described a method for measuring disease-causing mutations found only in the father's sperm, which provides a more accurate assessment of the risk of autism in future children. In other words, the risk of autism in offspring could be evaluated by means of quantifying the mosaicism of the male sperm. It has been suggested that *de novo* mutations that alter genes are involved in a range of at least 10% to 30% of autism cases, with a higher number of mutations in parents who are older at the time of conception. *De novo* mutations occur spontaneously in the sperm or eggs of the parents or during fertilization. Up to the time of this study's publication, when a mutation that could cause autism happened for the first time in a family, the likelihood that it could occur again in future descendants was unknown. So families had to make a decision with great uncertainty. These results suggest that genetic counseling would benefit from the addition of doing an evaluation of the mosaicism of the sperm. Nevertheless, we should keep in mind that this has to do with probabilities of risk and not of certainties.

## Alterations in neural pathways

Studies conducted in the field of neurosciences have served to elucidate the development of autism over time. To date, research has shown that aberrant brain activity and atypical brain morphology during infancy appear to be the basis for manifestation of autistic symptomatology. The greater brain growth in autism happens during a critical developmental age period, when the formation and connectivity of brain circuits are at their peak, at the most productive and optimal stage of synaptic activity (of connections between neurons). This growth can end up altering the formation of the typical brain connectivity necessary for optimal functioning of the neural pathways, a process that could eventually lead to autism.

It is worth dedicating a few paragraphs to understand how all this happens with a small review of **neurodevelopment**, that is, the different successive states that occur in the nervous system of the embryo, the fetus, and the first years of life until attaining certain complex brain structures.

The major milestones of neural development in the embryo include the birth and differentiation of neurons from stem cell precursors (neurogenesis); the migration of immature neurons from their birth places to their final position; the growth of axons from the neurons (cytoplasmic prolongations of neurons that drive electrical impulses) and the generation of synapses (connections between neurons) between these axons and their postsynaptic partners (the dendritic spines that receive the chemicals needed to generate a new electric impulse). Neurogenesis and neuronal proliferation take place throughout the prenatal stage; neuronal migration ranges from the first four weeks to eight or ten months; myelination and synaptogenesis (formation of synapses) begin in the prenatal period and last almost the entire life; finally, the neural pruning that, despite starting in early childhood, has its peak moment in adolescence. The following figure shows neurodevelopmental processes schematically in relation to embryonic and postnatal age.

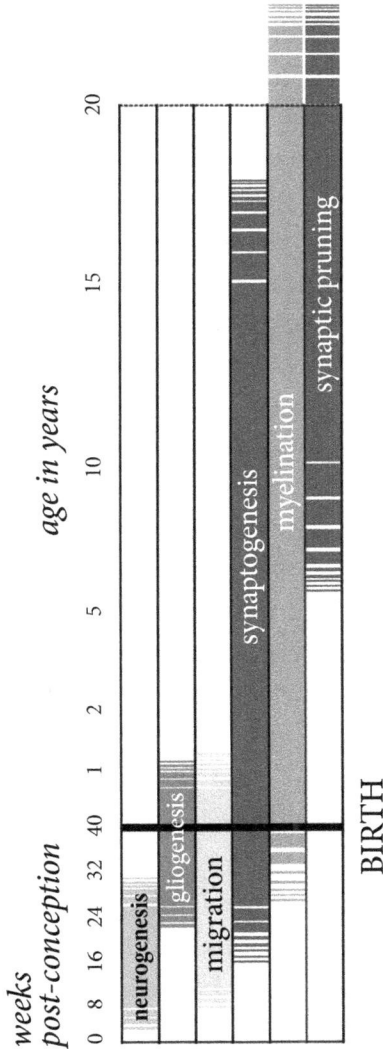

**Illustration 4.** Diagram of the different neurodevelopmental processes in relation to embryonic age and after birth. The length of the gray bars corresponds to the period during which the process is present, and the dashed lines are the beginning and end of the period where there is less activity.

The central nervous system derives from the ectoderm, the embryo's outermost layer of tissue. The neuroectoderm appears in the third week of human embryonic development and forms the neural plate on the dorsal side of the embryo. The neural plate is the source from where the majority of neurons and glial cells come. A groove forms along the neural plate and, during the fourth week of development, this folds over itself to give rise to the neural tube, which fills with cerebrospinal fluid. As the embryo develops, the anterior part of the neural tube forms three primary brain vesicles, which become the main anatomical regions of the brain: the forebrain (prosencephalon), the midbrain (mesencephalon) and the hindbrain (rhombencephalon). These simple, early vesicles expand and divide into the five secondary brain vesicles: the telencephalon (which will become the cerebral cortex and basal ganglia), the diencephalon (future thalamus and hypothalamus), the mesencephalon (where the colliculus will happen, which are the main nuclei of the auditory pathway), the metencephalon (from which the pons and cerebellum will form), and the myelencephalon (future spinal cord). Inside the neural tube, a central chamber filled with cerebrospinal fluid is formed, which is continuous from the telencephalon to the spinal cord and will form the ventricular system. That is, the neural tube gives rise to the brain and spinal cord. During this time, the walls of the neural tube contain neural stem cells that drive brain growth, as they divide thousands of times. Little by little, some of the cells stop dividing and differentiate into neurons and glial cells, which are the main cellular components of the central nervous system. The neuronal cell bodies make up the gray matter of the brain, while glial cells form the white matter. The newly-generated neurons migrate to different parts of the developing brain to self-organize into different brain structures. Once each neuron has reached its position, the axons and dendrites expand, which allow them to communicate with other neurons through synapses. Synaptic communication between neurons leads to the formation of functional neural circuits that intermediate in sensory and motor processing, and which form the basis for behavior. The following figure shows the stages of embryonic development:

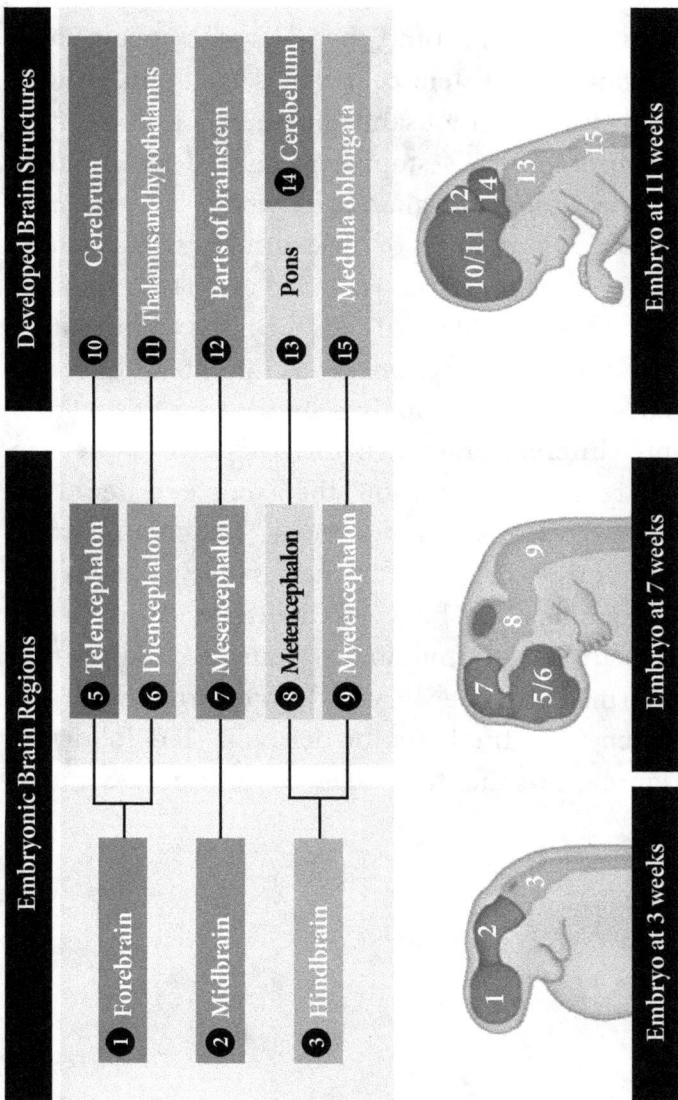

**Illustration 5.** Stages of embryonic development in relation to the brain regions that emerge from the neural tube and approximate age of the embryo. The different shades of gray correspond to the name and graphic representation of each brain region/structure.

Embryonic neurodevelopment processes are divided into two types: activity-independent mechanisms and activity-dependent mechanisms. The former are produced as wiring processes (from formation of nerve fibers) determined by genetic programs that develop within individual neurons. These processes include the differentiation, migration and orientation of the axon toward its initial target (to another neuron or different neurons). These processes are considered to be independent of neural activity and sensory experience. Once the axons reach their target areas, mechanisms come into play that are activity-dependent. Neural activity and sensory experience will mediate the formation of new synapses, as well as synaptic plasticity, which will be responsible for refining the nascent neural circuits. This differentiation between activity-independent and activity-dependent mechanisms helps to understand the changes that can occur in the prenatal period but also in the postnatal period, and the effects of the environment on the formation and development of the nervous system.

Some changes continue after birth, and some last a lifetime: The brain and the rest of the nervous system change with age, with a few early years of growth and progressive decline at the end of adult life. To sum up, the following table explains some of the brain changes and consequent changes in behavior at different stages of life.

| Developmental period | Brain changes | Behavior changes |
|---|---|---|
| **Early childhood** | The number of synapses increases rapidly.<br><br>The brain strengthens the connections it uses often and eliminates those it does not use. | The basis for brain function, memory and lifelong adaptability is established and grows.<br><br>A greater range of more complex actions is made possible, for example, raising the head, reaching an object, rolling, crawling, walking and running. |
| **Childhood** | Some parts of the temporal lobes continue to grow and reach their maximum volume.<br><br>Especially between the ages of 5 and 11, neural network connections increase in the areas of the frontal, parietal, and temporal lobes related to language and cognition. | The ability to understand, process and respond to social situations increases.<br><br>Between the ages of 5 and 11, many language and cognition milestones are reached. |
| **Adolescence** | Neural network connections in the frontal lobes continue to grow and strengthen.<br><br>The areas of the brain involved in reward, motivation and emotion also continue to develop. | The ability to reason about abstract concepts is developed.<br><br>Emotions increase in intensity and urgency. |
| **Youth** | Frontal lobe areas involved in target-oriented behavior mature.<br><br>White matter connections continue to increase. | The ability to control impulses and plan for them is controlled.<br><br>The brain can better integrate information (for example, when problems are solved). |

⟶

| Adulthood | Existing white matter connections are strengthened, allowing the brain to participate efficiently in more complex cognitive tasks. | Abstract reasoning, mathematical and spatial reasoning, and verbal capabilities increase. Optimism and social adaptation increase |
|---|---|---|
|  | In spite of neural networks being well established, the white matter in the temporal lobe continues to increase and the brain is able to reconnect already existing connections. |  |
| Old age | Some structures and regions of the brain are reduced. White matter decreases. | Complex mental processes may be negatively affected. Vocabulary and experience-based knowledge remain strong points. |
|  |  | Processing speed decreases and allowing additional time to complete tasks can be beneficial. |

**Table 3.** Main brain changes and their impact on behavior in different stages of life.

From what has been described so far you can understand the idea that, in a process as complex as neurodevelopment, there are many instances when alterations or variations can occur that can affect the formation of brain structures, the connection between neurons, the activity-dependent processes now outside the uterus, as well as many other genetically determined processes throughout personal maturation. What is most surprising is that, in the majority of cases, neurodevelopment ends up forming neurotypical brains with more similarities, and not so many differences, between them. And divergences in the form and functioning of the central nervous system only appear in a not very large percentage. Therefore, the pathogenesis of autism is not defined at a specific moment and does not lie in a single process, but is a cascade of altered processes that can occur both in the prenatal and postnatal stages, and throughout life.

Over the past two decades, many efforts have been made to determine the causes of autism as a developmental disorder. In this sense, the main findings have focused on alterations in neuronal migration. From a large range of highly-selective markers for subtypes of specific cells and a subset of candidate genes for autism, some very discrete pathological patches were detected that altered the laminar cytoarchitecture of the cerebral cortex (for example, the laminar structure of cortical neurons) as well as a disorganization in the majority of samples analyzed from prefrontal and temporal regions in children with autism. These patches were characterized by a decrease in the number of layer-specific or cell type-specific cells that are normally present in fully differentiated cortical neurons, forming amalgams of many undifferentiated cells. A possible explanation was found in neuronal migration, which would be altered by the presence of mutations in the genes expressed during this neurodevelopmental process. Although a transient increase in the number of cortical neurons during the second trimester of pregnancy is expected, this increase usually disappears at birth or during the months after birth, during which there is maturation in cortical laminar development and cortico-cortical and cortical-subcortical circuits (of the innermost structures of the brain). Nevertheless, the cause of this increase in the number of neurons in the prefrontal cortex in autism is unclear; this anomaly appears to be of prenatal origin and could cause an interruption in early cortical development.

Another process that has been investigated is synaptogenesis, and mutations have been found in different genes that had already been associated with autism symptoms, such as NRXN, NLGN, SHANK, TSC1/2, FMR1 and MECP2, which converge in common cell pathways that intersect in the synapses. These genes encode cell adhesion molecules, support proteins, and the proteins involved in synaptic transcription; protein synthesis and degradation, which affect various aspects of synapses; also, the formation and elimination of synapses, synaptic transmission and plasticity, thereby creating different or non-functional neural pathways. This suggests that the pathogenesis of autism can be attributed, at least in part, to a synaptic dysfunction. Variations have also been reported in polymorphisms of mTOR/Pl3K, which are mutations associated with abnormal synaptic and cellular growth.

These two processes could explain the earlier etiology of autism, as they occur mainly in the intrauterine period or in early childhood. However, the characteristics of autism vary in parallel with personal growth and maturation throughout life. For this reason, recent research has focused on the neural pruning that happens when the central nervous system is already formed and is boosted in adolescence. In other words, in normal development of the brain, an explosion of synapse formation occurs in childhood, especially in the cerebral cortex. Then, during late childhood and early adolescence (from 7 to 15 years), the synaptic density in the frontal cortex decreases by approximately 40%. These synaptic changes occur in the absence of significant neural losses and are accompanied by a reduction in expression of genes involved in axonal and synaptic functions. The continuous cortical thinning through synaptic pruning throughout childhood and adolescence reflects the maturity of the neural networks that are at the heart of behavioral changes in these periods. As has been seen, synapses are determined by many genes that show mutations in autism, and some researchers have hypothesized that people with autism may have more synapses. If synaptic pruning does not function properly (due to gene mutations or epigenetic changes in genetic expression) during development, the excessive synaptic connections are not eliminated and synaptic density will be higher than in the normal brain. A very relevant study in the journal *Neuron* in 2014 demonstrated the hypothesis of neural infra-pruning in autism (proposed by Chris Frith et al. in 2003). The study, done with post-mortem samples of brains from autistic people as well as mice, showed that an mTOR mutation could be one of the causes of autism, since the macroautophagic capacity of this gene was lost, leading to lesser neural pruning. In case studies with humans, diffusion tensor magnetic resonance imaging of the brain of autistic children has shown increased axons and myelination (with glial cells) among the areas closest to the brain as compared to the connections in more distant brain regions, which has been interpreted as an increase in connectivity. On a microstructural scale, increased synaptic densities of pyramidal neurons are observed in the temporal lobe of the brain of children and adults with autism in post-mortem studies. In addition, reduction in the density of the cortical column seen in the brains of adolescents in typical development does not occur in autistic individuals, again suggesting a deficit in synaptic pruning, at least at this stage of life.

The hypothesis of less synaptic pruning may help explain some of the most common symptoms of autism, such as hypersensitivity to noise, lights or social experiences, as well as epileptic seizures.

If there are too many synapses triggered at the same time, a person with autism is likely to experience an overload of noise and not be able to give an adequate brain response.

Disturbances in these neurodevelopmental processes have resulted in some neurobiological markers of autism. The main ones are an increase in brain volume in the first years of life, observable even before the age of 12 months in children later diagnosed with autism, both in gray and white matter, especially in temporal and frontal lobes and in subcortical areas such as the amygdalae (main structures related to the emotions). Until not long ago, increase in the cranial perimeter in early ages was seen as a characteristic finding of autism. However, this association is currently under discussion due to recent studies that found biases in the use of outdated growth tables and head circumference for population standards. In the direction of an increase in the size of some brain areas, brain neuroimaging studies found thickening of bilateral amygdalae at early ages related to joint attention impairments and with serious alterations in social communication at four and five years of age. Other longitudinal studies done in high-risk groups have described that aberrant development of white matter connections between 6 and 24 months preceded development of autism at 24 months. Using functional magnetic resonance imaging (fMRI), others have also found a lower correlation between the left and the right brain hemispheres in areas relevant to social communication.

Functional neuroimaging work has thrown light on the nature and pattern of brain activity and growth in newborns with autism. Specifically, reference studies by Courchesne et al. (2011) and Weigelt et al. (2012) detected growth patterns and notable changes in the cerebellar areas of the brain, even in the size of the cerebellar vermis, defined as a region of the brain responsible for motor control and cognitive functions. Precisely, children with autism showed atypical brain growth during the first and second years of life in the cerebellum and in cortical and limbic structures. These areas are responsible for the processing and use of cognitive, pragmatic, emotional, social, and higher-level language functions. Later research revealed that excessive brain growth is followed by an abnormal deceleration of the frontal brain areas (the most anterior and developed part of the human brain). These findings appear to provide evidence of the existence of abnormalities in autism, probably due to neuroanatomical lesions in multiple brain regions involving the number of cell bodies in the prefrontal cortex. Three years later, the Courchesne team analyzed the brain tissue of eleven children with autism and eleven healthy control subjects and found areas of immature cells and alterations in the layered structure, characteristic of the cerebral cortex in children with autism. This finding suggests that brains in autism have an excess of neurons because too many are formed, and perhaps also because too few are reduced in neural pruning. The impact of the intersection of life experiences and the cumulative effects of autistic social, cognitive and sensory deficiencies should be considered as an additional factor in the medium- and long-term of brain development at later ages.

In regard to functional studies, functional connectivity is a measure of the degree of synchronized activity between various brain regions, which is interpreted as a connection between brain areas. Over the past decade or so, a growing number of studies on autism have examined connectivity patterns with magnetic resonance while participants are not doing any mental activity (known as mind wandering). Some of these studies indicate that people with autism are characterized by insufficient connectivity between distant brain regions and a hyperconnectivity between neighboring ones; others show differences in connectivity within certain neural networks. In another study that focused on a neural network that is activated especially when we are doing nothing or daydreaming (default mode network), they found that connections between regions of this network in autistic brains were especially weak (these are regions that are distant from each other).

In accordance with this, the "connectivity theory" of autism states that in these brains communication between regions is atypical, in the sense that the specialized neuron bundles of neurotypical brains are not found. Instead, the connections would be more dispersed and not formed into bundles, resulting in less connectivity with remote areas and a lot of connectivity in nearby areas. In short, the autistic brain would be very branched but poorly arranged in bundles and, as such, with less connectivity between separate regions.

A related area of interest is connectivity of the prefrontal lobe and the amygdala. The few studies that have explicitly examined this connectivity in autism in the context of emotional regulation have shown inconsistent results. However, there are indeed numerous articles on abnormal medial prefrontal activity in autism that could affect emotional regulation, even though it is not known whether this is due to a hyperconnectivity or hypoconnectivity with the amygdala.

Various factors such as sex and age have been described that might influence patterns of functional connectivity. Also, several articles suggest that neural connectivity differs between children and adults with autism. For example, autistic children may have unusually strong connections in different brain networks; autistic adults usually show weaker connections in some networks. Entering puberty can reveal why their brains seem to change in this way and, once again, the alterations observed in neural pruning could be a valid explanation. The most valuable data comes from studies that monitor the time of connectivity within the same people. One of the few such studies suggests that connectivity between some brain networks increases from early adolescence to its end in typical people, but remains stable in autistic individuals. It has been proposed that lack of pruning maintains a brain that is very branched but which does not form specialized and well-connected bundles like in neurotypical brains.

Unfortunately, results from other studies disagree with the proposed patterns, and some find no difference between autism and the control brain. As studies become larger and more sophisticated, the number of divergent findings grows. In any case, one of the main reasons is the diversity in autism: each person with autism is different from all others, with a unique constellation of behaviors, experiences, and a specific genetics. It is not surprising, then, that individual connectivity patterns are also different. Conversely, there is indeed large agreement on the existence of peculiarities in the connectivity of autistic brains.

## Environmental factors

According to recent evidence, a range of up to 40% to 50% of variance in autism can be determined by environmental factors. Considerable progress has been made in understanding the different environmental risk factors, and the clearest evidence includes prior events and those that happened during birth, which will be seen below.

But it is highly unlikely that these factors alone cause autism. Rather, they may increase an individual's risk of developing autism when combined with genetic factors. In other cases, environmental factors related to problems during embryonic development have been suggested, in particular prenatal influences from alcohol, thalidomide —a nausea drug known to cause fetal malformations— and intrauterine exposure to viruses.

The study of environmental factors associated with autism has attracted interest from the National Institute of Environmental Health Sciences (NIEHS) in North America, which has a very generous budget from the government. Researchers funded by this organization have conducted several studies in recent years focusing on the interaction of genes and the environment, and which are references globally. The main conclusions that have been reached can be grouped by subjects:

- Air pollution: researchers found that early exposure to air pollution may be a risk factor for autism. Children of mothers living near a highway (at about 380 yards) and traffic-related pollution during the third trimester of pregnancy were twice as likely to develop autism. Another pollution-related finding was that boys and girls with a mutation in a gene called MET, combined with high levels of exposure to air pollution, showed an increased risk of developing autism.

- Prenatal conditions and maternal factors: problems with the mother's immune system, certain metabolic conditions, or inflammation during pregnancy appear to be related to an increased risk of autism in their sons and daughters. Some mothers of autistic people have antibodies or proteins in the body that fight infections, which can interfere with brain development in their children and could cause autism. Diseases such as diabetes or maternal obesity are associated with an increased chance of having a child with autism or other developmental disabilities, as well as having febrile episodes during pregnancy.

- Metals, pesticides and other pollutants: prenatal and early childhood exposure to heavy metals, such as mercury, lead or arsenic, presence in the blood of altered levels of essential metals such as zinc or manganese, and of pesticides and other pollutants have been studied by these researchers. Although different studies have been done focusing on mercury (very present in the fish we regularly eat in many parts of the world), they have found no association between this type of prenatal or dietary exposure (controlling the amount of fish eaten) and autism. On the other hand, a study of twins used baby teeth to determine and compare the levels of lead, manganese and zinc in children with autism with those of their respective twins without this condition. The autistic children had little manganese and zinc, metals that are essential for life, but conversely had higher levels of lead, a harmful metal during the specific developmental periods studied. However, this finding has still not been replicated. Nevertheless, researchers determined that altered cycles of zinc-copper that regulate the metabolism of metal in the body were aberrant in the people with autism included in the study. Finally, maternal exposure to insecticides during early pregnancy was associated with an increased risk of autism in their children. The role of other pollutants such as bisphenol A, phthalates, flame retardants and polychlorinated biphenyls in the development of autism has still not been determined.

- Nutrition: this field is the most controversial because of the disparity of studies and results that exist. However, studies funded by the NIEHS have discovered that taking vitamins during the prenatal period may help reduce the risk of autism. In addition, research suggests that taking vitamins and supplements may provide protective effects for people exposed to certain environmental pollutants during pregnancy. Specifically, women were less likely to have a child with autism if they took a daily prenatal vitamin during the three months prior to pregnancy and the first month of pregnancy, compared with women who did not take one. This finding was very evident in women and children with genetic variants that made them more susceptible to developing autism. Folic acid is a source of protection from prenatal vitamins. Women who took the recommended daily allowance during the first month of pregnancy had a reduced risk of having a child with autism, and pregnant mothers who took multivitamin products, with or without additional iron or folic acid, were less likely to have a child with autism and intellectual disability. A curious fact they demonstrated is that taking folic acid during early pregnancy could reduce the risk of having a child with autism in women with high exposure to air pollution and pesticides. Taking maternal prenatal vitamins during the first month of pregnancy may also reduce the recurrence of autism in siblings of children with autism in high-risk families.

However, over the last decade reviews have been published that question some of the results of the NIEHS, while others have consolidated their findings. In one of these reviews, published in *Molecular Autism* in 2017, it was suggested that varied environmental factors, such as vaccinations, maternal smoking, exposure to thimerosal (a preservative composed of ethylmercury and thiosalicylate used until 2001 in some vaccines), and assisted reproductive technologies would not be related to the risk of being autistic, while sufficient evidence was found about the link between some heavy metals (zinc and lead) and autism that warrant further research. In a review published in *The Lancet Psychiatry* in 2019, they showed that maternal factors, such as age and characteristics of metabolic syndrome, were associated with an increased risk of autism spectrum disorder. Although the use of antidepressants during pregnancy was also associated with this risk, when exposed and unexposed groups were compared, this association was affected by other confounding factors, taking into account that the use of antidepressants before pregnancy is also convincingly linked with an increased risk of autism spectrum disorder from the mother.

Be that as it may, the conclusion from the different authors of these reviews is that the mechanisms of association between environmental factors and autism are still unknown. They suggest that there may be less a cause-effect relationship, but rather that these factors have an influence and mediating effects with genes, oxidative stress, inflammation, hypoxia/ischemia processes, some endocrine impairments, alterations of neurotransmitters, and interference with signaling pathways.

# Autism through the Stages of Life

Autism is not a condition or disorder of childhood, but rather "lasts" a lifetime. The characteristics and difficulties of autism do not disappear with adolescence or when the person turns 18, even if for the education and health systems, and for society as a whole, it seems that way. While it is true that, for many children, the symptoms or characteristics of autism can improve with age and behavioral treatment, the reality is that during adolescence the manifestation of characteristics varies, with social, cognitive and emotional difficulties remaining; at this age, autistic people may become depressed, have a psychotic episode, or experience behavioral problems. For this reason, their treatment may need some modification as they reach adulthood. This is not strange after having reviewed the changes that take place in the brain throughout life. Likewise, these alterations, along with a nervous system that has had to grow and develop in an unfavorable environment, mean that autistic people continue to need services and supports as they mature and age. Everything will depend on the severity of the difficulties and one's own characteristics; some will be able to study, work successfully, and live independently, but the data indicates that most will need a supportive environment. If they do not have this, their lives will be a road full of difficulties and with devastating consequences.

## Before, during and after birth

It has already been mentioned that some prenatal factors may condition alterations during neurodevelopment or be involved in; these alterations result in a functional configuration of the brain. Autism cannot be detected before birth, as it is a multifactorial, polygenetic condition for which there is no diagnostic test. Up to now, autism in the prenatal stage has been a very interesting field of study, but not much more. How the person is affected at this stage cannot be measured and, in any case, progress is being made toward finding genetic markers that can determine the risk of having a child with autism after having confirmed the diagnosis in the first child or a previous one. With the increase in diagnoses in adults, some lines of research are beginning to analyze the offspring of autistic parents (with one or both parents), but at the moment there are no conclusive results.

A wide variety of possible postnatal factors for autism have been proposed, including gastrointestinal or immune system abnormalities, allergies and children's exposure to drugs, infections, certain foods, or heavy metals. Nevertheless, the evidence for these risk factors is anecdotal and has not been confirmed by reliable studies.

However, it is important to keep in mind that when a boy or girl has been diagnosed, many parents can recall behaviors and situations in which their child no longer seemed to function normally, such as showing little interest in other people or the way of interacting with others, especially with their companions at nursery school. Unfortunately, these signs are not sufficient to make a diagnosis in the first years of life and, for this reason, the diagnosis is made as of the age of three years or later, at the age of seven —on average— depending on whether language and intellectual capability are affected.

A large number of autistic boys and girls show developmental differences when they are babies, especially in their social and language skills. However, it is quite difficult to diagnose autism at these early ages. As some of those who will end up being diagnosed sit, crawl and walk on schedule, the less obvious differences in the development of body gestures, symbolic play, and social language go unnoticed.

## Childhood

This is the key moment for diagnosis of autism, especially in cases where there is no delay in language development or in intellectual capability —when there is a delay, the diagnosis can then be made before the age of three. Even so, in the first years of life some signs will have already been observed, which are summarized below:

- – little or no eye contact, or rather unusual eye contact; little response to parents' smile or other facial expressions; unusual use of the gaze, such as looking at objects from angles not often used;
- – not looking at objects or events that a parent is looking at or pointing out; not pointing to any object or event to get a parent to look at it; not carrying objects of personal interest to show them to their parents;
- – not having usual or appropriate facial expressions in each situation; difficulty perceiving what others may think or feel by

looking at their facial expressions;
- apparently not showing concern (empathy) for others; or having inadequate feelings toward the suffering of others; not knowing how to comfort someone;
- having difficulty making friends or having no interest in making them;
- starting to speak late (first words later than 16 months) if language is affected; not pointing things out to show need or to share things with others; or having very developed language at 18 months but without content (like repeating exactly what others say without understanding or sharing its meaning);
- not responding when called by name —which often makes people suspect deafness— but indeed responding to other sounds (such as a car horn or a cat's mewing);
- confusion among pronouns; they can refer to themselves as "you" and to others as "me";
- often showing no interest in communicating, not starting or continuing a conversation; or speaking in a non-reciprocal or unidirectional way;
- not showing a sociable smile;
- not using toys or other objects to represent people or real life in a simulated game;
- having good memory skills, especially for numbers, lyrics, songs, TV melodies, or a specific subject;

- showing stereotypical behaviors such as spinning, rocking, unusual finger gestures, walking on tiptoe for a long time, or flapping their arms in the air;
- presenting a need for routines, order, rituals; showing difficulties and discomfort with change or a transition from one activity to another;
- having obsessions with certain unusual or infrequent activities and doing them repeatedly during the day; playing with parts of toys rather than playing with the whole toy (for example, turning the wheels of a toy truck); or having hobbies experienced very intensely that interfere with their daily life;
- not feeling pain (or at least seeming that way); being very sensitive or having no sensitivity to odors, sounds, lights, textures, touch or taste (which can trigger restrictive eating behaviors).

These are just a few examples, which refer mainly to the areas of sociability, communication, behavior, language and sensory sensitivity. Each autistic person can show many of these signs or a few, that is, each person has their particular series of signs in early childhood. On a cognitive scale, it is difficult to detect any sign at this age. And regarding the emotional level, reactions of frustration to changes can be, as already explained, very exaggerated and with a high degree of irritability and aggression. Boy and girls with autism, when they have not yet been diagnosed, are often considered nervous, in the literal sense of the word.

The impact on life of this whole range of behaviors directly affects them in their adaptation to any environment where they develop, especially at home and at school. The manifestation of all these signs and symptoms is so heterogeneous and inconsistent that they delay diagnosis until later ages, especially if there is no effect on academics in the first school years, and if language, despite being peculiar, is, as has already been said, well developed. This means huge suffering in many families because it is difficult to understand what is happening.

Once the diagnosis is made and therapeutic interventions are started, the situation may improve, but we must not forget that autism cannot be cured. They are people with a different brain functioning that is not sufficiently prepared to live in an environment conceived and managed mainly by neurotypical people. This inability to fully decipher the world around them often makes school stressful for autistic people, and teachers often report that it is very difficult for them to meet the needs of students on the autism spectrum. As such, autistic individuals will always be in a situation of vulnerability that will not end when they move on to the next stage of life.

The dilemma at this vital stage revolves around whether to advocate for an inclusive school that respects and values the characteristics of autistic people, or whether special education centers are needed. It is not an easy question because the answer begins with an "it depends," and whether a father or mother is responding or if it is a teacher or educator.

Inclusive education is more than the fact that a student with a disability is accepted and integrated into a regular school, more than just an adaptation of the academic curriculum. Rather, it is more a value judgment; it is a way of improving quality of life, in which education can play a key role in providing the best opportunities and the same quality of resources to all the newcomers. It is a question of providing choices, being accommodating, offering resources and improving the education offered based on needs in order to favor inclusion and encourage a school that is effective and democratic, a school for everyone.

## Adolescence

Most adolescents with autism are thought to show less severe symptoms and behaviors as they become adults, according to some studies. But the reality is that not all autistic adolescents improve. Some, especially those with intellectual disability, may get worse. Many remain stable throughout their lives, even though it is true that about half, even with more disabling characteristics, see improvement over time, provided they have certain support available for their needs. Because improvement does not mean that autism disappears or decreases, but rather that it does not interfere so much in the person's daily functioning.

During puberty, adolescents experience changes in their bodies, focus more on who is "cool" and who isn't, and begin to experience sexual and romantic urges. These changes can be difficult for anyone. However, for boys and girls on the autism spectrum and their families, this stage can be especially complicated. The bodily changes that happen can be perceived as deeply alarming and may make them feel a certain amount of rejection. During puberty, they also begin to experience sexual impulses and crushes, which can be associated with difficulties getting closer to the person they like and, sometimes, sensory problems associated with autism that make sexual arousal cause anxiety or feelings of stress.

Adolescent boys and girls can begin to masturbate, a completely healthy and natural behavior in development. Nevertheless, unlike their neurotypical companions, they may not have the social awareness to know when and where it is appropriate to do so. In addition, different studies have described greater sexual diversity among autistic people, with higher percentages of homosexuality, bisexuality and transgender identity than in the general population. This can make the relationship with others and understanding of themselves even more complex.

And these bodily changes are in addition to the typical characteristics that have been mentioned thoroughly. They continue without social instincts, and this lack makes them vulnerable at a stage of life when being part of the group becomes something essential for development. Therapeutic intervention at this age is based on helping them learn to translate the —changing— norms that regulate social relationships, making the signs that come into play explicit, the reason to have relationships, and where doing things one way or another will take them, because they may not naturally understand this.

In adolescence, many autistic people experience a change from previous stages, in the sense that they lived more or less without apparent difficulties in childhood and, when they reach adolescence, autistic characteristics are manifested that are connected with a huge sense of unease and significant mental health problems (often with very diverse and not always accurate diagnoses). Or, conversely, there are individuals who were diagnosed in childhood and who, when they enter adolescence, see hyper- or hypo-sensitivity, stereotypy or some of their other characteristics decrease in frequency. There are other social difficulties that can become more evident, as demands from the environment are more complicated (interpersonal relationships are redefined during this period and become a mainstay in the maturation of any individual).

This period of searching and self-affirmation entails a certain distancing from parents, who have often been the only reference and support in the early stages of life. Without the safe place they have been able to establish with their parents, autistic adolescents may feel more alone and misunderstood than before. Despite wanting to have friends, their comments and inappropriate or defiant behaviors can lead to rejection, and even bullying and ostracism. This dysregulates them emotionally, and their emotional development is very negatively affected. When discussing autism in girls and women, the camouflaging strategies they do to be able to feel part of the group have been mentioned, resulting in an emotional exhaustion that can have consequences on their mental health in the short and long term. It is believed that the early female advantage allows autistic girls to seem like their neurotypical companions. However, this seems to decrease in adolescence, when physical, psychological and social changes create difficulties in maintaining friendships and understanding social conflicts.

Hence the importance of continuing with therapeutic intervention at this stage of life, because they need strategies and tools they can use in social situations. They need to be trained in certain aspects to be able to interact in an appropriate and autonomous way when they are adolescents, and also when they enter adult life.

However, external demands in adolescence are not only social. Studies or the first contact with working brings them fully into the world, where they no longer have the protection they had when they were children. Increased responsibilities are a source of stress, as quite often defects in neural pruning cause them to suffer from greater cognitive dysfunction and they may not be able to meet the requirements of their obligations with the cognitive resources they have. In adolescence, failing or dropping out of school are much more pronounced than in the previous stage. It is known that leaving secondary education or not getting a degree often creates serious problems to gain access to the labor market and remain there, as well as problems in social integration. Data from the 2016-2017 academic year collected in Catalonia showed that, of the 83% of autistic people schooled in ordinary schools, only 24% were enrolled in compulsory secondary education. A 2020 study done in the city of London found a very high rate of school absenteeism among secondary school students with autism (up to 43%). Along the same lines, the rate of school refusal behaviors —which are linked with long-term failure and dropping out— was six times higher in autistic adolescents without intellectual disability, according to a study done in Norway (Munkhaugen et al., 2017). Among other factors associated with this data, difficulties in detecting or accessing diagnosis in this educational stage has been identified, along with high vulnerability and the risk of failing at school or dropping out of the educational system prematurely; and also the transition from ordinary education to special education in order to complete primary education. One of the conclusions is that high schools are often not prepared to take in students who have a greater need for support and, even less, having autism associated with intellectual disability, which contributes to the decline in compulsory schooling among young people with autism.

The transition to the world of work can be even more dramatic, and little attention is paid to what happens after childhood, even though the adult population is larger than that of children. For all adults and their families, employment is a major concern. However, this concern is much greater for families with members on the autism spectrum. The lack of secure employment means that financial demands are very large not only for autistic adults and their parents, but that this also adds costs associated with additional care, such as the system for assistance and expenditures on public health, which becomes a huge economic burden for nations. Unemployment levels are disproportionately high in autistic adults, with the best estimates indicating that 80% of autistic adults not having language and intellectual development affected have been unable to find long-term employment. And this figure is even worse for those who are more highly affected.

Administrations are not capable of responding to needs in this stage of life and tend to be more specifically focused on intellectual disability, but not on other types of difficulties. Protected jobs are very scarce and tax breaks for companies usually end up in the wastebasket. In light of the need, various local initiatives have been created, from foundations and private associations to certain companies that consider autism to be an asset for the company rather than a disability. One such company, though not the only example, is Specialisterne, a Danish social innovator company with branches in different countries. At Specialisterne, autism is the norm rather than the exception among the employees. Other examples can be found, including some companies in the banking and pharmaceutical sectors, but resources are currently very limited and best practices are not shared or agreed upon. In other countries, such as the United Kingdom, what is known as the Autism Employment Alliance has been created, which aims to raise awareness in society on autism after childhood, to promote legislation in favor of employing autistic people, and to work on developing support for autistic adults as well as business owners.

## Adulthood

Awareness of autism in adults is progressively growing in recent years, reflecting an increase in diagnoses as well as an understanding in certain sectors of society that, also in later stages of life, a diagnosis can offer important benefits and relief. Often, diagnoses of autism that are made after adolescence happen in cases where it has been possible to function fairly well in terms of adaptation to the environment (but which does not exclude having suffered incomprehension, isolation, emotional distress and other problems). In cases where the autistic person has not had good adaptation, it is likely that the comorbidities of autism have been diagnosed but not autism itself, such as avoidant personality disorder, obsessive-compulsive disorder, major depressive disorder, eating disorder or language disorder, and that treatment also has not been effective enough. These diagnoses come, in part, from widespread ignorance of the signs and symptoms of autism in adults, especially in those who were never evaluated or diagnosed during childhood.

The most common symptoms of autism in adults, and which confuse specialists when making the diagnosis, include difficulty interpreting what others think or feel, problems interpreting facial expressions, body language or social signs, and difficulties regulating emotions. They can also show difficulty in maintaining a conversation and are prone to monologues on their preferred subjects, with restricted and special interests; they tend to do repetitive or routine (but not stereotypy) behaviors, ranging from food restrictions to rituals for doing any daily activity. They like to maintain daily routines and can explode if there are changes in them. They have executive difficulties that interfere greatly in their daily life (they usually need visual and auditory supports to function and respond to the schedules in adult life). In short, they have an autistic repertoire very similar to the one in the previous stages of life, but in a certain way adapted to the moment in which they are living.

At this stage of life, autistic women can imitate social standards better than some autistic men; they often describe how they adapt to people or imitate them. An autistic woman may show a wider range of emotions with her face and voice. They may be able to adopt social standards quite well, but they find it exhausting and stressful. The greater emotivity in relationships between women can seem really overwhelming and unpleasant to them, so they often gravitate toward male friendships. The intense and restricted interests of women are often more socially relevant pastimes: they can become volunteers or sign up for NGOs and help with environmental causes. This often masks autistic traits. As already mentioned, another characteristic of autism in women is that it is more closely associated with eating disorders than it is in men. Studies also suggest that women with autism who are diagnosed with anorexia benefit less from treatment than non-autistic patients. These women's dietary restrictions could be for nutritional reasons or they may be repetitive food profiles owing to sensory problems or because they crave this repetition. Because the eating disorder is the most critical and obvious condition, autism is often overlooked. Furthermore, one of the risks for autistic women is that they are taken advantage of in social relationships. A study by Bargiela et al. reported an incidence of sexual abuse in autistic women of more than 60%, with half of these abuses happening with the regular partner.

During adulthood, meltdowns or shutdowns continue to happen. Situations that other people may find easy to deal with or solve can be really difficult for autistic people, as has been widely described, to the point of causing a meltdown. In the words of Sarinah O'Donoghue, a BBC Scotland contributor who is autistic, "The meltdown seems as if my body is trying to escape the chaos in my mind. I feel upset, I cry and scream to distract myself from the intense noises inside me, which I can't control." This feeling of "melting" (hence the English expression) usually affects the body and mind, to the point of becoming physically painful and psychologically distressing, all at once. The most common signs of a meltdown include head-hitting, kicking, pacing, rocking, hyperventilation, being unable to communicate and completely withdrawing into themself —some adults may flap their arms, but it is not as common. All these behaviors are methods of coping and to try to calm down.

In some environments, meltdowns can be very disruptive, which is why it is good to know what they are and why they are happening. There are many factors that can cause them, but perhaps the most frequent are moments of intensified sensory processing. Sensitivity to light, odors, heat, sounds, taste and touch is increased. An example of this may be the increased awareness of feeling clothing on the skin. Underlying feelings of anxiety, stress, ambivalence or incomprehension can make the sensory overload more severe.

To conclude this section, it is worth adding a few comments about being an autistic father or mother. On the one hand, there is the decision to have children, since, as has been widely commented, autism is hereditary. On the other hand, there is what this maternity or paternity is like. People with genetic changes associated with autism usually inherit a higher risk of being autistic, but the condition is not inherited in and of itself. Autism spectrum disorder is a complex and genetically heterogeneous disorder that has made it difficult to identify the etiological factors of each person and, consequently, to provide genetic counseling for families at risk. However, in recent decades notable advances in knowledge on the genetic aspects of autism based on genetic and molecular research, as well as the development of new molecular diagnostic tools, have substantially changed this scenario. Today it is estimated that, through currently available molecular tests, a possible underlying genetic cause can be identified in nearly 25% of cases. Combined with clinical evaluation, assessment of prenatal history, and investigation of other physiological aspects, an etiologic explanation of the disease can be found in approximately 30% to 40% of cases. Taking into account current knowledge of the genetic architecture of autism spectrum disorder, which has contributed to more precise genetic advice or counseling, and the potential benefits that etiological research can provide to users and families, molecular genetic research has become increasingly important. Despite all these advances, the proportion of families who consult a genetic counselor is still very small. First, because there are not many experts in this field and, second, because of a lack of knowledge about autism. Genetic counseling can benefit these families enormously, as it can provide them with suitable information that can influence reproductive decisions and even, in some cases, guide interventions. This is good for families where autism is a *de novo* mutation as well as for those where the parents are autistic or have first-degree autistic relatives.

There are parents of autistic people who are neurotypical, others where one or both parents are autistic, and others, between 17 and 23%, who have what is known as **broad autism phenotype**, that is, although they do not meet the characteristics necessary for a diagnosis of autism, they indeed show some of them. Many mothers and fathers realize they have autism when they begin to investigate the characteristics of their son or daughter. Being an autistic child or adult is difficult because of all that has been mentioned previously. But what can be more difficult is to be an autistic mother and, even more so, to be an autistic mother of autistic children. They do not have it easy because of their own autistic traits, which can make raising children difficult, and also because many autistic mothers hide their condition out of fear that administrations and social services will take their children by misinterpreting their autistic traits as potentially dangerous for the child. There is a certain belief that these women cannot be good mothers because of the negative connotations of their condition. It is the unassailable barrier of stigma that they may encounter to access services or seek support among family members or friends, who from the very start may reject or be very critical of their maternity. A 2020 study led by Baron-Cohen found that mothers with autism were more likely to have had additional psychological problems, including prepartum or postpartum depression, and they pointed out greater difficulties in areas such as multitasking or in coping with household responsibilities and creating social opportunities for their child; which are explained, in turn, by executive dysfunction, social communication difficulties, and emotional dysregulation, as well as due to changes in routines and lack of sleep. Women participating in the study reported more often that they felt misunderstood by professionals and showed more anxiety, higher risk for selective mutism, and lack of knowledge about what details were appropriate to share with the professionals. It was also more common for them to experience maternity as an isolating experience, to worry that others would criticize how they were raising their children, or to feel unable to turn to others for help. Despite these difficulties, however, autistic mothers showed that they acted in the interests of their children, putting their needs first, as there were not more cases of neglect, of any kind, detected with them than there were with non-autistic mothers. In short, autistic mothers face unique challenges, and the stigma associated with their condition can aggravate the difficulties related to raising children. Greater understanding and acceptance are therefore needed among the people interacting with autistic mothers.

## Old age

For many autistic adults, the golden years of old age are tarnished by overall poor health, economic problems or poverty and, in some cases, homelessness. Their situation reveals enormous gaps in personal care and in the aid and support earmarked for these ages. In fact, you could say that autism in old age is a completely forgotten fact, because many autistic people who reach advanced ages may not have been diagnosed with autism and, conversely, may have received many other psychiatric diagnoses —if they end up receiving any at all. This implies not receiving good treatment, a circumstance that entails endless consequences for not having been properly diagnosed during most of their life.

Some recent research suggests that older autistic people are more at risk for a wide range of physical and mental health conditions, such as diabetes, depression and heart disease. They are also about 2.5 times more likely to die prematurely. The reasons for these very serious statistics can range from the diagnostic errors already mentioned, missed medical visits and incorrect dosages of medicine, to a lifetime of social alterations and discrimination. In a 2011 study, researchers determined that 14 out of 141 residents in a psychiatric hospital in Pennsylvania had undiagnosed autism, and that all but two had been misdiagnosed with schizophrenia. Many others have been diagnosed with lifelong intellectual disability, with the consequent limitation of development opportunities, which is further exacerbated in old age. Diagnosing adults with autism is difficult because tests are designed primarily for children; details about early life are also requested, which for older adults whose parents have died may no longer be available, or the person is unable to express them in the right terms.

That is, without a diagnosis, elderly autistic people cannot access many services that can help them to secure housing and medical care. And even after a diagnosis, those with low incomes and no one who takes care of them can lose their housing and be moved to group homes, where insufficient care and support can lead to untreated medical problems. The loss of parents and other caregivers can also break an emotional and practical support structure, leading to deterioration in mental and physical health. Surely many of the reasons why they end up with more health problems are because they do not get the support they need to manage health care in adulthood. A significant fact is that social work and welfare resources are not adapted when the person to which they are directed is autistic. To take one example, proposing to a person who has social difficulties, hypersensitivity to strong odors, and does not understand certain unwritten rules that they go to a shelter will probably not be of much help.

Autistic grandparents are likely to have health problems for the same reasons that young autistic people do. Autism shares genetic roots with conditions such as schizophrenia, attention deficit disorder and hyperactivity, and with various types of cancer, and evidence also suggests a biological link to Parkinson's disease. Some features of autism can also imply health risks, which can become worse over time. For example, unusual food preferences and a tendency to be sedentary, both common among autistic people, may end up taking a toll. Medication can also have undesirable effects, as it is often prescribed for mistaken diagnoses and is not effective, as well as due to side effects. People with autism can take antipsychotic drugs that can cause weight gain, high blood pressure, and an increased risk of diabetes and heart disease. Likewise, these diseases can lead to other problems such as persistent sleep apnea, which can be common in autistic people and if it persists can, in turn, increase the risk of diabetes and heart conditions.

But perhaps what is most responsible for all these consequences in the last stage of life is the society in which we live, which is not very friendly when it comes to differences. To survive, many autistic people camouflage their characteristics, trying to act like neurotypical people all their lives, and this continued masking can end up being very stressful. Therefore, without proper support, autistic people over time experience burnout, a phenomenon characterized by chronic exhaustion, loss of skills, and even suicidal thoughts and behaviors. Social isolation can aggravate these health problems. Loneliness, feelings of alienation, and a sense of rejection are common among elderly autistic people and can lead to depression.

A more accurate diagnosis, the access to care and adequate support are essential to improving the prospects for this group of abandoned older people, according to experts, although there are few studies to support these observations. And with the greater awareness we are starting to have, we should learn. In fact, there is no systematic research on autism in people over the age of 65 and thus the nature of the problems is unknown. But with the aging of the population and recognition of a higher prevalence of autism than previously thought, it seems the path is beginning to take shape.

# Chapter 5

# Living and Autism

The demands of living as an autistic person or with an autistic person are huge and often involve high levels of stress. Parents must learn how to deal with certain behaviors and follow treatments while planning their children's future; siblings and other family members may feel embarrassed or not understand certain situations; couples may feel overwhelmed; and friends may need time away to be able to maintain the friendship. Recognizing the challenges involved and preparing for them is thus essential for everyone involved.

To begin with, it may be necessary to clarify that autism is not the result of poor child rearing by the parents; autistic people are not rebellious or spoiled, nor do they have behavioral problems; the vast majority of people with autism are not wise or talented (though many examples on television present them like this); and we must keep in mind that autistic people have feelings and emotions. With these few premises, it is easier to establish and implement some strategies and guidelines for living autism well.

## Schooling

In the educational world, regardless of the level of disability, the teaching program for an autistic person must be based on the unique needs of this person. To help determine what type of learning environment is best, an Individualized Education Program (IEP) should be developed. This should include some clear and measurable goals to be able to assess the child's progress and be reviewed annually or, if necessary, more often. Ideally, all areas of the student's development should be addressed, including academic achievements, objectives for social and adaptive behavior, and the development of fine and gross motor skills. Development of communication skills (fundamental in autism) should be an essential component of the IEP. Finally, it is important that the IEP not only address areas of need, but also explain ways to take advantage of strengths in specific subjects or skills. Autistic children can be educated in partially or fully integrated classrooms with neurotypical classmates, in specialized classrooms within regular school, or in specialized schools for students with special needs. Wherever it may be, a highly-structured educational environment is required, with appropriate support and adaptations in line with individual needs. The educational program should be based on the person's interests and use visual cues to accompany the instructions given. When necessary, other services, such as occupational or language therapy, need to be incorporated to deal with problems having to do with development of motor skills and sensory integration. The key elements in creating a suitable educational environment for autistic students are for teachers to set high expectations for each one and encourage interaction among classmates; for both special educators and ordinary teachers to feel involved in the process; instructions should be individualized while at the same time shared with the entire class; support services, whenever possible, should be done within the ordinary classroom to facilitate generalization and avoid stigmatization (sometimes these end up benefiting other students without special needs), assuming that everyone can acquire skills if instruction is modified to help them succeed. In short, it is about having a collaborative approach, which includes regular and special educators, administrators and school personnel as well as parents.

Most member states of the European Union have policies guaranteeing the right to a free education without discrimination. However, some states, such as Poland, do not have a specific strategy for autism, while others (for example, the United Kingdom, France and Spain) do indeed have policies specifically designed for autistic people. Despite the differences between states, they all seek to achieve the same goal: an inclusive education for autistic children that leads to the development of their full potential.

The change from preschool to primary school and from this stage to secondary school deserves a separate chapter. There are changes in the buildings and surroundings, the school and then the high school are larger, the facilities can be confusing. Students do not know the teachers and, in turn, new teachers may not know anything about the autistic student. New classmates may not be used to having a classmate that is autistic or has some other condition that makes them different. Thus, the transition needs to be planned. Unfortunately, this is not done as often as would be desired, nor are the resources available to do so. Therefore, from home or in collaboration with teachers, whenever possible, a series of actions may be done that can help in making these transitions through the educational stages (extracted from free materials offered by the Autism Society of the United States):

- Write a social story or a series of stories to help the student prepare for the change.
- Allow the student to make as many visits as needed to the new school.
- Practice the route to walk to classes with the building empty or with very few people.
- Identify important areas, such as a safe haven, the bus stop, study hall, restrooms, the cafeteria and the gym.
- Practice how to put things in their backpack, and opening and closing their locker.
- Help the student understand school rules (including unwritten ones): lining up when they are younger, respecting the cafeteria line in high school, not making noises during class, etc.
- Practice behavior scripts so the student knows where and how to ask for help. For example, learning to detect when they are getting nervous and asking to go to a quiet place to calm down.
- Prepare the student to understand that each teacher has different rules and procedures, so they must therefore be flexible with each one's rules.
- Look for a system that helps the student keep their notes and other school materials organized.
- Request training sessions to orient them spatially and move around the campus at the

IEP meeting.
- Have help in the classroom, such as a recording device or notes on the board, so that tasks and homework are documented.
- Request a laptop or other technological support for the student who has little writing ability.
- Have some trusted classmates so the autistic student does not enter the school alone or have to go alone to different places in the school building.

## Work

In order to enter the work sphere, good "transition" planning can help autistic people make an easier shift from high school or the educational environment to adulthood. The general or ordinary educational community has long been working on the transition from school to work, with more or less success; teaching plans plot out more academic paths to reach the university or work-focused ones to do training modules, and most undergraduate degrees have pre-work programs or internships in the final years. Unfortunately, despite years of compulsory transition planning, interest in preparing autistic students for real life has instead been rather negligible, leading to high drop-out rates, high unemployment (according to data collected in the United Kingdom in 2019, only 16% of autistic people had a stable job), low wages, few work options, limited relationships and restricted life options. And not only this. Some drop out of school without being prepared to handle simple daily routines such as paying bills, balancing the budget and maintaining an orderly living environment. This bleak perspective demands that those involved in the education of young autistic people must have effective transition planning that is done seriously and systematically.

Surprisingly, some countries, such as the United States, have regulations dictating that students who receive Individualized Education Programs (IEPs) during schooling must have transition services as of age 16. According to Osborn and Wilcox (1992), transition planning must fulfill several important functions, such as introducing the family and student into the services system for adults, determining the support required by the student to live, work and participate in the community as an adult, and identifying deficiencies and inadequacies in the services system for adults. All this allows members of the transition team to advocate for more suitable services, provide information to service providers for adults about individual needs so they do not assume when planning services and implementing programs that all people with disabilities have identical needs, and to provide critical information to determine the correct objectives with which parents and educators can best guide development of the skills needed for a smooth transition. For the time being, it is utopian to think about common regulations from our administrations, but until work is done on this, the dramatic consequences that have been described will continue to exist and will prevent people with autism from living well.

In this regard, one of the fundamental problems is the quota of vacancies for people with recognized disabilities, but also access to unprotected jobs for autistic people who do not have any degree of recognized disability. Usually, because of their characteristics, they cannot work on a rigid schedule, or the conditions required exceed their sensory, adaptive and productive capabilities. This means they have to change jobs, must go on numerous job interviews (without having the necessary social tools, which creates frustration so they end up not showing up) and, in the worst case, they end up not working at all, or working in little known or lower paid places.

In the meantime, some small gestures can be tried at a local and personal level, such as involving the person in curricular options that can teach them other important life skills, such as cooking, repairing items and managing personal finances; encouraging autistic young people to participate in after-school activities, school clubs, and other social events to help them build a support network that will make access to employment easier later on.

While they are still in school, the autistic person should be supported in doing apprenticeship programs, so they can have positions as volunteers or other options that allow them to gain experience in a real work environment. They can be helped in starting to build a resume, tapping into their tastes and preferences, and doing this in various formats using video and computers, which make their own competences more visible. It is necessary to gradually prepare them for the nuances and social demands of the job, and make this one of the objectives of psychological therapies: talking and making clear what behaviors can clearly run counter to the rules of most work environments, learning to control behaviors that can disturb co-workers and lead to dismissal, etc.; in short, show and put into practice appropriate behaviors in specific workplaces in as natural an environment as possible.

Among these appropriate behaviors, it is important to remember to include hygiene and dress standards appropriate for specific work environments and instructions on social interactions on suitable topics, which can help them have spontaneous conversations in the office and during work-related discussions. Initial preparation for the job can avoid unnecessary difficulties and promote long-term success, particularly in terms of possible reactions to their unusual behaviors, or in the more than likely comparison with other colleagues in terms of efficiency. This is why it is good to identify a person within the work environment who can be a "mentor," someone the person can easily go to for help, advice or whatever is needed. It would also be ideal for the working environment to be favorable to autism (the previously mentioned autism friendly environment), which means creating an environment that reduces the negative effects of sensory differences and improves positive effects since, as already noted, autistic people perceive the world very differently than other people do.

When looking at work options —although often there will not be much choice— safe and efficient means of transportation must be found. If public transportation is chosen, the routes, timetables and alternatives must be considered in case there is any alteration. Availability of transportation is essential for independence.

## Social environment and leisure

In the social environment, the demands that autistic people face are more changeable and uncontrolled. Due to social unease and suffering, autistic people can become anxious and withdraw socially, even if they wish to have friendships and social contact. This is a lifelong problem. In most cases their participation in settings outside the family or primary school/ high school is virtually nil, such as in public spaces, entertainment facilities or places belonging to friends and the extended family. This means that these people are not exposed to a wide range of appropriate activities like the ones their non-autistic counterparts experience, such as sports, mobility, cultural events, shopping, work or socializing with friends. Participation, defined by the World Health Organization as involvement in life situations, is understood as "participating in or performing meaningful activities in occupational and social roles while being present in these." Participation is considered both as attendance, understood as "being there," and involvement, which includes elements of commitment, motivation, persistence, social connection and emotional levels within the environment. Therefore, for autistic people, participation is a point of contact for learning and for social development, as it is intertwined with family, peers, public life and society, which form part of their environment. In the case of adolescents, this is even more crucial for their socialization and the transition to adult life. If there is no participation during adolescence, you can hardly expect that it will be present in adulthood or old age. Unfortunately, support from the environment for participation in the community by autistic people is rather low, which means that adolescents, especially, avoid participatory experiences because they feel pressured by their efforts to balance the idea of "being different" with the need to "fit in." Constant pressure becomes a heavy weight and prevents involvement with the peer group. The lack of these appropriate experiences can end up having a negative impact on job independence and relationships in adulthood. In addition, it can adversely affect health and quality of life.

However unworkable it may seem, autism associations and foundations strive to facilitate attendance by autistic young people at activities outside the setting that is most familiar to them. The problem is that not everyone has access and not all families are aware of these initiatives or these are not sufficiently available. Again, the public administration does not provide the necessary resources for universal assistance to autistic people, and it is not that it is impossible to do so —associations and foundations show us that it can be done— but rather that given the difficulty, decisions are made that do not improve the quality of life for people who do not fit into the available public resources (such as day centers or jobs with support designed for people with intellectual disability or serious mental illness).

## Family

Living with autism affects the family and people close to the autistic person, whether there is a diagnosis or not —in the latter case the stress of not knowing what is happening can be a huge burden. Raising autistic children with autistic mothers has already been mentioned, but in many cases parents do not have this condition. Most neurotypical parents, family members and caregivers focus their efforts on helping the autistic person, even if they do not know how to do it, which affects marriages, other children or relatives, work, finances, and personal relationships and responsibilities. The difficulties and needs of an autistic person complicate family relationships, especially with siblings.

When there are one or more people on the autism spectrum in a family, stressors are added to their daily life. There is the physical stress of preparing meals, bathing, homework, shopping, schedules —quite common in all families— and the psychological stress resulting from conflicts between parents and children —also usual— to which factors related to the autistic way of doing things and behaving are added. The fact that autistic people show communication problems and rigidity, which make it difficult for them to express their basic needs or desires in a typical way, means that parents or those close to them are often playing a guessing game. This lack of communication and understanding, along with the rest of the daily difficulties, makes everyone involved feel frustrated. The autistic person's frustration can lead to aggressive or self-injurious behaviors that threaten their safety and the safety of other family members (for example, siblings). Stereotypical and compulsive behaviors worry parents, as these are odd and interfere with functioning and learning. If the person has difficulties in social skills, this increases concern and stress in those living with them. People who do not have adequate skills in regard to leisure often require constant structure, which is virtually impossible in environments that are out of the family's control.

In many families there are additional challenges related to sleeping or with meals. Many parents often end up giving up after years of trying to get their child to sleep at night or eat a wide variety of foods. All these problems and behaviors are physically and emotionally exhausting for families and the others living in the home. Inappropriate or maladaptive behaviors can prevent families from attending events or activities together. Not being able to do things together can affect the marriage, the relationship within the couple, or the relationship with peers. In addition, spouses often cannot spend time alone due to the extreme demands on parenting and lack of qualified personnel to monitor an autistic person when they are absent.

When they decide or manage to do community activities with the people close to them, other people may stare, make comments, or not understand whatever mishap or behavior that might happen. As a result of these experiences, the people who have come along can often feel uncomfortable. This makes vacations or trips especially difficult. Not being able to socialize or have relationships with others can mean, for parents or those living with people on the autism spectrum, feelings of isolation and rejection from society.

Raising and educating an autistic son or daughter requires extraordinary demands on parents as individuals and on the family as a whole. Among these demands, the main one is to meet all their needs, for which there are not enough hours in the day. Specifically, the time it takes to meet the needs of an autistic family member may leave parents with little time for their other children. Many parents believe that, despite doing their best for their autistic child, they always struggle to respond better to the needs of the entire family. They often report that, although their own life as an individual might be "on hold" and the couple may understand the need to make sacrifices for the benefit of their autistic son or daughter, few parents are willing to make the same effort toward the other children in the family. As a result, there is continuous tension between the needs of the autistic child and those of the others. And it would be a very serious mistake to fall into a negative —and superfluous— criticism of these parents. What is needed is to be aware that there are a number of special demands for these siblings, and that learning to manage them will make their childhood easier and will teach them skills that will make them more effective and resilient adults. The best teachers to demonstrate these adaptive skills are precisely the mothers and fathers. The advice and relationship models these parents give their children during childhood and adolescence will be of use to them immediately and in all the following years.

For all these reasons, having the diagnosis and access to treatment can help reduce the stress that comes from not understanding and not knowing what to do. Those closest as well as the autistic person themself can help their other family members by letting them know about autism and the complications it presents, understanding the challenges that siblings face and helping them to cope with them, and getting participation from the extended family to create a network of help and understanding. Attending mutual support groups (groups of non-professional people who meet to share a physical, psychological or social health problem or a social risk situation, in order to provide mutual support and share information with an eye toward achieving personal or social change) can help in this understanding and to not feel so alone.

Common sense tells us —and research supports the idea— that family and friends need to understand what autism is. It is important that people close to autism are aware of it and that the information they get is appropriate and verified. From early childhood, they need explanations that help them understand the behaviors of the autistic person they care about. One of the keys to success is to remember that we all need to be continuously informed about autism. Most people can use the words they hear here or there, but they may not fully understand their meaning. For this reason, books like this one are so needed!

# Chapter 6

# Strategies for Daily Life

This chapter has been very much in demand by many people who live closely with autism and who do not hesitate to act, research, read and develop strategies to be able to live well, or at least much better. The reality is that it is difficult to find materials or sources that pull together some clues for daily life at home and in the surrounding environment. There is indeed a good amount of documentation for professionals, educators and support people, but this scarcely translates into clues for surviving daily coexistence, given the difficulties involved in autism. One possible explanation is that it is not very easy to put all the things that might be useful into writing or in a document, or because autism is so heterogeneous, watertight recipes work for some cases, but not others. Be that as it may, after dozens of talks, following are some proposals —in no case exhaustive— about what can be done from autism and for autism in daily life.

Organization of the strategies presented is based on "the other characteristics of autism," as they are the behaviors and traits that most alter good daily functioning. In addition, therapeutic interventions are already usually focused on the core symptoms of autism. These strategies are useful notwithstanding the other treatments being followed with professionals, whether individual or group psychotherapeutic sessions or appropriate drug prescriptions. They are based on this broader concept that has been described in the previous chapters, taking into account neuroscientific advances and the sociological and cultural conception of autism.

## Emotion regulation

Emotion regulation is terminology used generally to describe a person's ability to manage an emotional experience and respond to it effectively. People unconsciously use emotion regulation strategies to deal with the many difficult situations that come up throughout the day. A person with good emotion regulation skills may notice when they are emotionally "overloaded," may think about the consequences of their response, and can continue to do what they are doing without losing sight of their goal while feeling negative emotions. Autistic people do not have this well-developed ability, as has been described above, and therefore explode when faced with a wide variety of situations; they experience negative emotions for longer, have little resistance to frustration, and are blocked by emotional explosions; and they also have mood swings.

The first thing it is necessary to work on is to identify and label the emotions. It is clear that these tasks need to be done when the person is well and in a good mood. You can create a chart or table of emotional levels. Each person can establish labels, both visual —with simplified faces or colors— and with the written language they need. One example would be to put 'feeling good,' 'a little annoyed,' 'annoyed' and 'very annoyed.' The last row can be given to the meltdown. Once you know what can trigger a meltdown, you must think of ways to minimize this trigger. Each autistic person is different, but sensory differences, changes in routine, anxiety and communication difficulties are common triggers. The graphic should have two columns, with the emotional levels in the left-hand column, while in the other column will be written "I feel like this when...". Finally, the rows will be left blank to fill them in.

| Emotional state | I feel like this when… |
|:---:|:---|
| ☺ Good | |
| 😐 A little annoyed | |
| 🙁 Annoyed/sad | |
| 😠 Very annoyed/ angry | |
| 😖 Overwhelmed | |

Table 4. Example of a table to identify emotions.

Second, how to assign these emotions to everyday situations and determine whether they are appropriate or not must be taught with the help of a trusted person.

Third, and this is a very important point, you have to talk about each reaction and find out which would be the most appropriate and also the healthiest.

Finally, healthy coping strategies must be learned and put into practice, such as taking deep breaths (there are mobile apps that are very useful with this), count to 20, ask for help, talk to a friend, find a compromise solution (not you, not me), get away from the situation, think of something nice or a happy memory, etc. But it should also be remembered that these strategies might not work during a meltdown. In these more extreme cases, the best strategy is to let a reasonable amount of time pass and as much as possible avoid getting to this last box by minimizing the triggers, as has been mentioned above. Other types of emotion regulation techniques are sensory strategies, which can easily be done at home. This has to do with finding activities that stimulate the main senses as well as proprioception (self-perception) and sense of movement, such as listening to music, chewing gum, hugging yourself, jumping, hitting a pillow, rocking, doing tactile pressure activities with objects (pushing a wall), massages, etc.

In the case of a meltdown, there are a series of actions that the people near the person suffering from this can do. First of all is safety, so it is necessary to find a space with minimal stimulation. It is also useful to have some sort of object that provides a feeling of calm (carrying this with you can be of great help) and can work for stimming. Third, and this is difficult for neurotypical people, it is necessary to decrease requirements and demands, as the meltdown comes from cognitive, sensory and emotional overload. And fourth, you must leave time for the reaction to happen. You should never try to stop behavior with violence or brusque movements, unless the person is physically harming themself or others.

Emotion regulation can be practiced and end up having very positive effects, but at the same time you must show respect and understanding of negative thoughts and feelings. At times it is necessary to take a step back and consider why one feels a certain way, what has caused this or what it is that cannot be communicated at this moment. A good way for them to learn is by trying to identify the first signs of distress and intervene before the negative behavior escalates. The way of perceiving these first signs can be strange, such as noting itching in your eyes, having a stomach ache, noticing pressure in your head, etc., so it is necessary to have a very open mind to be able to associate this with negative emotions. Maintaining direct and ongoing communication with therapists or support people is a strategy that should continue to be done.

# Reducing anxiety

Anxiety is a very common characteristic of autism, but it can manifest itself in different ways in each person. Learning to detect anxiety symptoms is, once again, a very good strategy to be able to cope with it. A series of questions can be considered to determine if you are anxious, such as: "Am I worried about something —although I don't know what it is— all day?", "Do I feel nervous, apprehensive or like I'm at my limit?", "Am I experiencing unpleasant physical sensations, such as butterflies in my stomach, tense muscles, dizziness, feeling like I can't sit still, etc.?", "Is it difficult for me to relax and disconnect?", etc. It is clear that in cases of non-verbal autism or with intellectual disability, requesting that they ask themselves these questions can be difficult or even impossible. In these circumstances, it will be important for the people close to the autistic person to learn to detect these symptoms so they can put strategies into practice to gradually reduce the anxiety levels. Some of these observable signs of anxiety can be quickened breathing, unexplained stomachaches or chest pains, palpitations, sweating, muscle tension when touched, trembling, or having difficulty concentrating.

Anxiety increases negative thoughts which, in turn, increase physical anxiety symptoms. This creates a vicious circle, which is what we want to break. Even if these thoughts, catastrophic and against oneself, are not verbalized, the kinds of ideas that suddenly come up have to do with worry and discomfort, which gradually increase.

Strategies to reduce anxiety in autism are very similar to those for emotion regulation, but in this case relaxation and breathing techniques play a more important role. Trying to do alternative thinking strategies or cognitive therapies —very common in treating anxiety in other conditions— may not be a good option for autistic people, and using physical rather than cognitive strategies might be better. Changing activity and environment, doing physical exercise (running or walking), practicing diaphragmatic breathing, etc., are techniques that help break the vicious cycle of anxiety.

People often pick up the habit of avoiding situations that make them feel anxious. Unfortunately, this can make the problem worse. The longer and more often something is avoided, the more intimidating it becomes. Moreover, if situations that cause anxiety are always avoided, it is more difficult to learn how to manage them. And so you progressively lose self-confidence.

## Do sleep hygiene

Good sleep means falling asleep, staying asleep during the night, and that this sleep is good quality. All people, including autistic ones, need a good night's sleep for growth, development and learning.

Typical tips for good sleep hygiene generally are:

– Establish a bedtime routine.
– Establish regular and suitable schedules for rest in each stage of life.
– Associate the bed and bedding with a restful sleep.
– Establish a safe and comfortable sleep environment.
– Avoid caffeine, screens and emotional excitement before going to sleep.

But often, despite making every effort, problems with falling asleep, getting up frequently during the night, or having a lot of difficulty getting up in the morning are problems that are not resolved with these rules. This is because autistic people do not understand these circumstances nor feel like they are their own. As much as they try common strategies, they are hard-pressed to assimilate them.

There may be stimuli that interfere with autistic people's sleep but go unnoticed by neurotypical ones.

Keeping in mind the sensory and cognitive processing of autism can help to detect the situations and environmental factors that make it difficult for them to fall asleep and stay sleep, and to try solutions that are based on this understanding. Some examples include:

- Noises that are unexpected or difficult to locate and interpret can be an annoyance that makes it hard for them to fall asleep. Using noise-canceling headphones can prevent unavoidable noises from interfering with sleep. Helping to detect the source of the noise and interpret it properly can also be helpful.
- The presence of lights when they wake up during the night can upset them. Making sure the room is dark or with points of light that are well placed to prevent them from noticing other lights while sleeping or when they wake up during the night is an easy strategy to reduce interference.
- Bedding and nightclothes they do not find comfortable. Tactile hypersensitivity can trigger discomfort that is difficult to communicate. Using natural fabrics without rigid textures, having favorite garments that make them feel calm, can help encourage them to go to bed.
- Emotional excitement is usually a response that arises without an immediate cause but because of a memory or situation that is remembered *a posteriori*. Thus, it is difficult to control that this does not happen right before going to sleep. Having a relaxing fidget toy near the bed can help decrease the excitement and make it easier to sleep.

– Sensitivity to odors can also interfere, so using hand lotion with a familiar and pleasant smell can also lighten the emotional overload that prevents them from falling asleep.

All these aspects must be worked on beforehand, whether it is an autistic adult without intellectual disability —in which case they can prepare things themselves— or if they are autistic children or young people, who can get help from their parents. What is important is that they adapt to the sensory processing itself.

In terms of cognitive processing, strategies would be linked to understanding why you should sleep and why it is important that sleep be sufficiently restful. This is a perspective that is being introduced into the guidelines for sleep hygiene from the metacognitive dimension, of thinking about oneself. Here you can make records of how the day is spent after you have slept well and after you have slept poorly —understanding the definition of restful sleep. It is also interesting that daytime activities help to make a good differentiation between day and night. If you do similar activities at night (such as using the computer or exercising or eating a lot), falling asleep can be more complicated. Changing the clothes you slept in when you get up also lets you make this distinction from the day-night cycle.

Adolescence is a time when sleep problems can get worse or appear for the first time, as all teenagers experience a schedule change when they get past puberty. What is known as the "internal clock" changes and, suddenly, they do not feel tired or sleepy when they go to bed, nor can they wake up as early. Instead of trying to get the teen to go to bed when they are not sleepy, it is often more useful to delay bedtime by half an hour or an hour, keeping in mind that they need about eight to nine hours of sleep. If the rest of the people living in the house also establish similar schedules, it will be easier for them to adapt to the new habit. It will also help if there is no more than one hour of difference between workdays and weekends for bedtime and wake-up time.

## Controlling disruptive behaviors

Disruptive behaviors in autism are probably the most worrying for autistic people as well as their family or friends, as they can interfere a lot in daily life, leading to undesirable and problematic consequences. Forms of disruptive behavior that can occur in autistic people include self-injurious behaviors (for example, hand-biting, head-hitting, punching, scratching until they bleed, etc.), assaults and destruction of objects or property, among others. Disruptive verbal behaviors such as insults, hurtful comments, or disparaging language can also happen. In these cases, support from others is needed to manage this behavior; you cannot ask the person doing it to also be the one to deal with it. The "management" of these behaviors is often done with specialists, but as they may appear frequently and in any situation, some clues and strategies are needed to avoid serious consequences from them.

The way to deal with these behaviors in daily life should not be to punish or demoralize the autistic person —although this is quite often the automatic response these behaviors elicit. Rather, it is about setting limits and communicating expectations in a stimulating and comprehensive way.

In the childhood and adolescent stages, discipline is one of the most important tools that can be used to show that we trust them and are concerned about them. Discipline should focus on correcting problematic actions, showing what is right and wrong, what is acceptable and what is not. The benefits of discipline are the same whether the people have special needs or not. For discipline to work, it is essential to act consistently in all situations, have information about the condition of the autistic person, define expectations of what the discipline wants to achieve, to use rewards —not necessarily material ones, to offer praise, smiles, etc.— explaining the consequences that derive from the discipline, and to always use it by means of clear and simple messages.

To be disciplined with children and adolescents is to have trust in them and to be convinced that they can learn and put into practice more adapted behaviors without negative consequences.

On the other hand, understanding why disruptive behaviors occur in autism may help to deal with them in a more positive way. First, think about what role this disruptive behavior plays from a non-autistic perspective: Do they want to get away from an unwanted task or situation?; conversely, do they want to get something they don't have at that moment?; are they demanding attention?, etc. Disruptive behavior must also be considered from an autistic perspective. By describing disruptive behaviors as flight from an "unwanted task," it is implied that these behaviors are the choice of a willing and spoiled intellect. For many autistic individuals, disruptive behaviors are based on fear or pain. A task can be unknown, and the discomfort it can cause is not easy to understand or manage if one does not experience it. The "unwanted task" can also be a known task that is painful or confusing, even if the people who help the individual do not see it like this. For example, a person who has a meltdown while getting ready in the morning before leaving home and has difficulty processing all the changes that happen quickly, and who also feels great discomfort from the friction of their clothes against their body. What should be kept in mind, therefore, is that inappropriate behaviors are difficult to change because they are functional, they serve a purpose, so it is necessary to work on finding a way that is appropriate and non-disruptive to express the discomfort. This is the basis of the Positive Behavior Support (PBS) technique, which tries to address problematic behavior caused by environmental factors or lack of sufficient skills by reducing this behavior in order to improve the person's quality of life, under the principle that the function of disruptive behavior is legitimate, but not the way it is expressed.

On the other hand, it has been suggested that some autistic behaviors, such as stimming, stereotypy and, in people who are hyposensitive (that is, they require more stimulation to feel sensations) behaviors such as excessive moving to give themself added movement, making buzzing sounds or other noises to add auditory stimuli to their surroundings, or getting excited and enthralled by decorative details, smells or textures around them, would be a way to seek constant pleasure and well-being. Cutting off these behaviors can create great frustration for them and can ultimately turn them into more disruptive and problematic behaviors.

Therefore, when an autistic person has disruptive behavior because they do not want to do something they are being asked to do or because one of their "moments of pleasure" is being ruptured, we must try to break the task down into smaller parts, provide a break for self-stimulation and then continue with each part of the task, provided that the problematic behaviors are controlled. In the event that the disruptive behavior is due to a demand for attention or interaction (for example, showing problematic behavior when the other person is speaking on the phone or pays attention to something else), you should not respond and they should be told that only when asked properly will attention be paid to them. If the disruptive behavior manages to be controlled, then it is a good idea for the interlocutor to pay attention as soon as possible and with an explanation, if necessary, of why attention was not paid immediately. Using timers to establish a time-out period is often useful. The most important thing is to ignore inappropriate behaviors.

It may also be that the disruptive behaviors have no clear function or, at least, they cannot easily be related to any of the above cases and are more serious (significant aggression or self-injury). If so, these strategies may not work and it will be necessary to get urgent help from professionals.

## Training executive functions

As mentioned above, many autistic people have difficulties in cognitive functioning and, in particular, in executive functions. The problems are mainly with skills such as planning, staying organized, controlling impulses and sequencing information. At the same time, they may have other cognitive functions that are not altered and even have much better functioning than that of the general population. Some of these functions are memory, extraordinary perceptive capacity, attention to details and patterns and, because many other functions are not automated, there may be a higher awareness of processes (in the case of people without intellectual disability). Although now it is difficult to find professionals who focus their interventions on these aspects, neuroscientific advances and the changing perspective on neurodevelopment are gradually contributing to expanding the field of intervention in autism. One example is the very promising results in cognitive rehabilitation of executive functions in autism, but which have not for the moment been translated to healthcare practice.

In the meantime, the day-to-day strategies that can be done to improve executive function consist in using strengths to cope with difficulties, which in turn can help build a stronger foundation for social and communication skills. Although our executive functioning is a highly complex system, effective interventions need not be. Some easy tips can be:

- Make lists of tasks or activities to be performed.
- Set time limits for tasks (timers are very useful).
- Make schedules in which each day is planned.

- Make the reason for each task and the time it takes explicit (telling yourself this out loud can help).
- Explore different ways of learning; often repetition by the parents of how to do something does not help to learn it, and it is more useful to find a logical explanation from the autistic person's perspective.
- Establish routines with clear steps and remember them out loud if necessary.
- Use rewards (in children and adolescents) and self-rewards (in adults) that give a sense of fulfillment and self-confidence —they should not necessarily be material, a "I really did that well" type of recognition may be enough.
- Use of self-instructions or written instructions; these techniques are based on how language is normally used to self-regulate behavior. They can make posters or write on a board the instructions that are more difficult to incorporate for doing whatever type of daily task.

Apart from simple (or not so simple) strategies, there are those who require a little more involvement from the people close to them (parents, partners, others living in the house, etc.). This is what is known as "making frontal lobes of the other," as the autistic brain has the frontal pathways for control much more branched and less specialized, as was described earlier, which leads to these cognitive and executive difficulties.

Use of (good) visual cues: Visual cues is one of the techniques that has the most amount of evidence in the treatment of autism. Here it is about using it to improve sequencing of tasks to be done —for example, before leaving home in the morning. Photos, diagrams with steps, clues left as reminders (leave the keys on the table near the door, put the bag by the door, etc.), visible and audible alarms to perform the tasks, can be used. Touching the visual cues with a finger at the moment the action has been done often helps.

Use of gestures to accompany the actions: In relation to the use of cues, there is a large amount of evidence on the role of gestures in executive functioning. A particularly interesting finding from this line of research is that neurotypical children who used many gestures performed better in cognitive tasks than children who did not use accompanying gestures. Associating a gesture with each action would be like putting a check mark when it has been done, which strengthens learning. Because of the underlying basic deficits in social communication, many autistic people have difficulty using and understanding gestures. By directly helping in teaching and encouraging the use of gestures, parents, partners or others can help them improve their ability to solve problems, reach goals, keep information in their working memory, and be flexible when changing tasks. For people with greater cognitive impairment or intellectual disability, touching and pointing to the morning routine on the visual map is a way to gesticulate. If the person looks at the visual map and says the steps out loud without touching the picture, you must ask them to show you by pointing to them. Should the autistic person need it, you can take their hand to help them advance in the process.

Plan before, perform after: To be able to establish this order of plan before and perform after, there is a previous step, which is to know what the finished product is like (for example, to be ready in the morning at a specific time) and what it entails (the positive consequences: arrive on time at work / school). This is the only way to determine the logical sequence of tasks to be performed. Talking about the finished product and achieving the goal is a big help; you can talk about how the person will feel when they are ready on time and ready for the day, but also about the discomfort that comes with not achieving this. This step helps to develop future thinking, and also to make preparations. Then you need to work backwards, thinking about all the steps that will have to be taken, writing them down or putting in visual cues and, when the task is done, putting a check mark on the list, touching the objects or saying things out loud.

In short, it is about training one's independence, following the premise according to which the help received is of the type 'do with, not for; do less, not more,' to the point in which external help is no longer needed and one trusts themself and the plan before, perform after system. The impact of these three strategies can be increased through social stories to help guide the steps of any type of routine. Although social stories are very common in interventions with autistic children, using them with adults also helps for organizing tasks. For example, "When I wake up, I get out of bed and go to the bathroom. I go back to the bedroom and put on my clothes for the day."

Finally, a strategy that combines different executive aspects and helps manage time and control the restricted behaviors that often interfere with daily functioning is the use of planning matrices. These are tables that include restricted activities or behaviors, and alternatives are progressively added to work on flexibility without increasing discomfort. The goal is to become aware of rigid and restricted thinking and behaviors, of the time they take up in daily life and how this interferes in other aspects.

| Interest/ meal/ activity | Time spent per day /number of times | What have I stopped doing | How I feel 1: bad - 4: very good | Alternative |
|---|---|---|---|---|
| **Train websites** | 4 hours | I have not studied | 3 | Dedicate 2 hours to it |
| **Pasta with sauce** | 5 times/ week | Eat healthy | 4 | Eat salad 2 days |
| ... | ... | ... | ... | ... |

**Table 5.** Example of a planning matrix to progressively change restricted activities or behaviors.

Let's turn to Pete Wharmby to look at the most important of these strategies. Wharmby is an autistic teacher, writer, tutor and father, and has a Twitter account with more than 32,000 followers (@commaficionado). As a summary, following are some clues and strategies so that non-autistic people understand how to interact with autistic people:

1. Have a quiet area to allow "emotional decompression" when needed.
2. Give very clear and unambiguous instructions.
3. Don't expect them to react in a way you would expect, because they often show their emotions in very different ways.
4. Don't assume they are incapable of thought and feeling if they are non-verbal, nor that they are incapable of communicating in other ways.
5. Don't expect autistic children to stop being autistic when they grow up. This simply does not happen.
6. Don't force them to wear particular clothing if they show a nearly visceral reaction to it; its texture or fit might be causing significant discomfort and unhappiness.
7. Don't be upset if they don't wish to socialize with us, as they often have considerable difficulties with social skills. However, try to do it, as it's nice to at least have the opportunity to do so.
8. Check in on autistic people from time to time while with them. Don't be upset, however, if

they don't respond quickly —all socializing is stressful and many tend to be forgetful of others and disorganized.

9. Don't use jokes or insulting humor with autistic people, unless there is sufficient trust or you know they won't be offended.

10. Remember all autistic people have a very different experience of autism —it's a huge list of traits. That is, any combination is possible and should be taken carefully.

11. Don't force them to make phone calls. Often they don't know how to hold a conversation and it can be very stressful for them.

12. Don't force eye contact. Many autistic people find eye contact way too intimate and emotionally draining, but it doesn't mean they aren't listening to us!

13. Let them stim. These movements, sounds and behaviors are ideal for regulating stress levels and are absolutely vital. If these aren't allowed, there is greater risk of harming themself or others.

14. Let them speak and listen to their special interests from time to time. It may be a bit exhausting, but they need to have "safe" listeners and will appreciate it very much.

15. Let them play with their toys however they want (at any age!).

16. If an autistic person forgets something, don't be too harsh with them. It's hard to remember things when just surviving is complicated.

17. Remember that many autistic people have comorbid conditions. We must be sensitive to this aspect and assume nothing.
18. Don't infantilize autistic people. They are not big kids, they are adults with a special way of thinking and acting.
19. Don't spread misinformation about autism and condemn it when you see it.
20. Pay attention to how we address them. Many autistic people have gender diverse identities, or do not feel classifiable.
21. Don't assume that verbal autistic people are "high functioning." They may be good at certain things, but you don't know to what extent daily life is difficult for them.
22. Don't use 'autism' or 'autistic' as if it were an insult or a taboo, nor use euphemisms.
23. Give opportunities to autistic people if possible, they are often more creative due to how their brain works. Doing this can bring about very positive changes.
24. If an autistic person does a job, they should be paid like a non-autistic person would.
25. Don't force an autistic person to do something they're uncomfortable with unless you know that pushing them can help them. You have no idea how scared they may be in that situation.
26. Let autistic people follow their routine as much as you possibly can. It helps them immeasurably and doesn't usually cost anything to let them do so.

27. If an autistic person has a meltdown or shutdown, give them space and don't judge them. Be kind and let them rest afterwards.

28. Don't tell anyone who says they are autistic that they're not autistic. First, because you don't know enough about autism; second, your objection is probably based on incorrect stereotypes; and third, it's rude.

29. Give enough processing time to answer when you ask them something, even if it seems like an easy question.

30. And, above all, follow autistic accounts on Twitter, Facebook, YouTube, etc. They are a great source of first-hand information!

# Thinking about autism

Autism raises questions that go beyond basic assumptions about what is different or what is normal, or what is genius and what is deviation. Autism, among other neurological or neurodiverse conditions, opens an especially provocative debate about existing societal models and what should be changed in order to live better. This has to do with whether all individuals should be forced to conform to social norms established by the majority, as well as whether these rules need to be gradually adapted and made more flexible, understandable and useful for all people.

The great disparity in conceptualization is not unique to autism. The truth is that neither psychology nor psychiatry have ever been unequivocally associated with the natural sciences, or minimally this has been a more recent attempt, along with the birth of neuroscience. In fact, some still consider psychiatry to not be a medical specialization like the others, as it is not organic. This was the reason why, for a long time, mental illnesses, psychological conditions or organic psychosyndromes were considered in different ways and based on peculiar references, and often with little consensus. I could have taken advantage of this book to, once again, complain about attempts by psychologists or psychiatrists to distance social and cultural elements from their research objects in order to move closer to the world of science, which frankly I found quite tempting. But it was not about that. Rather, it has to do with trying to explain the path —and the factors that have defined it— of the classification of psychiatric and psychological diagnoses and, specifically, in this case, of autism. The aim is to try to discover the story behind the changing borders and taxonomies of what is called scientific in the study of psychopathology in this century. The story deals with certain unstable intellectual and disciplinary spaces that seem to require more fluid and optimal relationships with epistemology, interdisciplinary studies, science and social aspects. Combining all these elements is not easy, but with perseverance some milestones have been reached that have allowed us to understand this phenomenon a little better.

However, we will always be navigating between two perspectives or ways of understanding autism. On the one hand, the view that refers to autism as a dispersed and disaggregated phenomenon, something that can only be understood from multiple dimensions or by means of different levels of understanding (from genes, cognition, behavior, brain anatomy, sensory levels, time, environment and life experience), which are not necessarily connected to each other or, at least, not in an obvious way. And on the other, the view that is based on scientific research in many fields that mixes, connects, creates, intertwines or traces the different sources of knowledge.

Neurosciences, in the broadest sense of the term, have revealed what the autistic brain is like, how it works, and how it can explain the wide range of characteristics that are grouped in autism. Functional deficiencies stem from basic and fundamental social, communicative, emotional and cognitive deficits that cause problems for learning, perception, organization, comprehension, generalization and, ultimately, brain overload. These difficulties lead to significant problems when it comes to dealing with new situations, as well as with those situations that require generalization of knowledge by means of environments. Even for autistic people with greater cognitive ability, problems with generalization of knowledge in real-life situations are a source of considerable impairment, even though these functional difficulties are often not considered defining characteristics. This is why the model that has emerged from the neurosciences, again in the broadest sense, could be a good scenario for understanding autism and making it visible in the twenty-first century.

No one is immune to the changes brought about by the global COVID-19 pandemic. For adults on the autism spectrum, the loss of routines and expectations is especially damaging and often leads to seemingly insurmountable anxiety. For individuals of any age across the autism spectrum, support from the family and members of the health care team is essential to facilitate the transition from established routines to new ones at school, at home, and at work. Autistic adults should explore strength-based tactics to stay in touch with others, improve self-regulation, and plan alternative ways to meet needs, achieve goals and find suggestions for self-care. The goal of this quick immersion is to have provided fairly in-depth knowledge about autism that is useful as a basis to propose practical solutions that are easy to implement (but difficult to achieve) in order to cope and thrive as an autistic person, both during this unstable time and in any situation.

# Glossary

**Arousal**: Physiological and psychological state in which a person is awake or reactive to stimuli, with a quickened heart rate and high blood pressure, and with a condition of sensory alert, mobility and readiness to respond.

**Gaussian distribution or bell curve**: Normal distribution was described by Abraham de Moivre and widely used by mathematician Carl Friedrich Gauss. Any human phenomenon follows this distribution in which the majority of individuals with the characteristic are concentrated in the middle part of the bell and on both sides the frequency with which the phenomenon occurs decreases in an asymptotic manner. In the author's book *Mundos Invisibles (Invisible Worlds)*, there is a detailed explanation of the normal curve

**Allostatic load**: The "wear and tear on the body" that accumulates as an individual is exposed to repeated or chronic stress and tensions.

**Social or functional disability**: a limiting situation that can have its origin in health, if basic needs are not covered, in a lack of skills or minimum competences, a lack of support, stigma, in the family environment, an inaccessible environment, in a cultural environment that puts obstacles in the way, etc.

**Broad autism phenotype**: There is considerable evidence that some of the cognitive and behavioral characteristics associated with autism are also present in first-degree relatives who are not autistic. For example, compared with individuals with no known family history of ASD, non-autistic parents and siblings of autistic individuals have shown higher levels of autistic-like traits, worse language skills and more social communication difficulties.

**Symbolic interactionism**: Psychosocial theory as well as a methodological framework in which human behavior and thought are the result of social interaction, specifically, the exchange of meanings. Historically, it is interpreted as fighting on two fronts: psychological reductionism and structural (biological) determinism, focusing on the capabilities of the actors, the action and the interaction conceived as processes. Source: Wikipedia (ca.wikipedia.org).

**Meltdown (or shutdown):** Exaggerated emotional reaction that has different manifestations such as being irritated, lashing out at others, sobbing uncontrollably, shouting, developing all kinds of unhealthy (even self-destructive) behaviors, while a shutdown is an internalized distress that cannot be expressed externally.

**Neurodevelopment:** Development of the nervous system from the moment of conception through various biological processes. It is also understood as the capacity of the living being to develop the brain pathways responsible for brain functioning to be able to learn, focus, develop memories and social skills, etc.; in short, to adapt to the environment.

**Neurodiversity:** School of thought defending that brain differences are normal phenomena, rather than deficits, within human variability. The idea of neurodiversity can have advantages for people with differences in learning and brain processing. It arose with the idea of reducing the stigma associated with psychiatric and neurodevelopmental disorders, and mental health conditions in general.

**Stimming:** Any behavior that consists of repetitive actions or movements characteristic of people with developmental disorders, most typically those on the autism spectrum. It is a type of sensory self-stimulation.

# Further Reading

American Psychiatric Association (2013). *Diagnostic and Statistical Manual of Mental Disorders*, Fifth Edition. Arlington, VA: American Psychiatric Association.

BARGIELA, S.; STEWARD, R.; MANDY, W. (2016). "The Experiences of Late-diagnosed Women with Autism Spectrum Conditions: An Investigation of the Female Autism Phenotype." *Journal of Autism and Developmental Disorders*, no. 46(10), p. 3281-3294.

BARON-COHEN, S. *et al.* (2013). "Do girls with anorexia nervosa have elevated autistic traits?" *Molecular Autism*, no. 4, p. 24.

BARON-COHEN, S.; LESLIE, AM; FRITH, U. (1985). "Does the autistic child have a "theory of mind"?" *Cognition*, no. 21(1), p. 37-46.

BARON-COHEN, S. (2002). "The extreme male brain theory of autism." *Trends in Cognitive Science*, no. 6(6), p. 248-254.

BREUSS, M.W.; ANTAKI, D.; GEORGE, R.D. et al. (2020). "Autism risk in offspring can be assessed through quantification of male sperm mosaicism." *Nature Medicine*, no. 26, p. 143-150.

CHARMAN, T.; PICKLES, A.; SIMONOFF, E.; CHANDLER, S.; LOUCAS, T.; BAIRD G. (2011). "IQ in children with autism spectrum disorders: data from the Special Needs and Autism Project (SNAP)." *Psychological Medicine*, no. 41(3), 619-627.

COURCHESNE, E. *et al.* (2011). "Neuron number and size in prefrontal cortex of children with autism." *JAMA Psychiatry*, no. 306(18), p. 2001-2010.

COURCHESNE, E.; PRAMPARO, T.; GAZESTANI, VH et al. (2019). "The ASD Living Biology: from cell proliferation to clinical phenotype." *Molecular Psychiatry*, no. 24, p. 88-107.

DAMASIO, AR; MAURER, RG. (1978). "A Neurological Model for Childhood Autism." *Archives of Neurology*, no. 35(12), p. 777-786.

DWORZYNSKI, K. et al. (2012). "How different are girls and boys above and below the diagnostic threshold for autism spectrum disorders?" *Journal of the American Academy of Child and Adolescent Psychiatry*, no. 51(8), p. 788-797.

SHEFFER, E. (2018). *Asperger's Children: The Origins of Autism in Nazi Vienna*. New York: W. W. Norton and Company.

FITZGERALD, D. (2017). *Tracing autism: uncertainty, ambiguity, and the affective labor of neuroscience.* London: University of Washington Press.

FRITH, C. (2003). "What do imaging studies tell us about the neural basis of autism?" *Novartis Foundation Symposium*, no. 251, p. 149-166; discussion p. 166-176, 281-297.

FRITH, U. (2003). *Autism: Explaining the Enigma* (2nd ed.). Oxford: Blackwell Publishing.

International Classification of Functioning, Disability and Health (ICF). https://www.who.int/standards/classifications/international-classification-of-functioning-disability-and-health

JAHROMI, L.; BRYCE, CI; SWANSON, J. (2013). "The importance of self-regulation for the school and peer engagement of children with high-functioning autism." *Research in Autism Spectrum Disorders*, no. 7(2), p. 235-246.

KIM, JY et al. (2019). "Environmental risk factors and biomarkers for autism spectrum disorder: an umbrella review of the evidence." *The Lancet Psychiatry*, no. 6(7), p. 590-600.

LAI et al. (2016). "Quantifying and exploring camouflaging in men and women with autism." *Autism*, no. 21(6), p. 690-702.

MANOUILENKO, I.; BEJEROT, S. (2015) "Sukhareva-Prior to Asperger and Kanner." *Nordic Journal of Psychiatry*, no. 69(6), p. 1761-1764.

MODABBERNIA, A.; VELTHORST, E.; REICHENBERG, A. (2017). "Environmental risk factors for autism: an evidence-based review of systematic reviews and meta-analyses." *Molecular Autism*, no. 8, p. 13-29.

MUNKHAUGEN, EK; GJEVIK, E.; PRIPP, AH; SPONHEIM, E.; DISETH, TH. (2017). "School refusal behavior: Are children and adolescents with autism spectrum disorders at a higher risk?" *Research in Autism Spectrum Disorders*, no. 41-42, p. 31-38.

OZONOFF, S.; PENNINGTON, B.; ROGERS, S. (1991). "Executive Function Deficits in High-Functioning Autistic Individuals: Relationship to Theory of Mind." *Journal of Child Psychology and Psychiatry*, no. 32(7), p. 1081-1105.

PAULA, I. (2015). *La Ansiedad en el Autismo: Comprenderla y Tratarla*. Barcelona: Alianza Editorial.

ROLESKA, M. et al. (2018). "Autism and the right to education in the EU: Policy mapping and scoping review of the United Kingdom, France, Poland and Spain." *PLoS ONE*, no. 13(8) e0202336. https://doi.org/10.1371/ journal.pone.0202336

SAMSON, A. et al. (2013). "Emotion regulation in children and adolescents with autism spectrum disorder." *Autism Research*, no. 8(1), p. 1-10.

SCHROEDER, INICIAL et al. (2010). "The neurobiology of autism: Theoretical Applications." *Research in Autism Spectrum Disorders*, no. 4(4), p. 555-564.

SCHULZ, S.; STEVENSON, R. (2018). "Sensory hypersensitivity predicts repetitive behaviours in autistic and typically-developing children." *Autism*, no. 23(4), p. 1028-1041.

SILBERMAN, S.; NEUROTRIBES (2015). *The Legacy of Autism and the Future of Neurodiversity.* New York: Avery, an imprint of Penguin Random House.

SIMPSON, JN (2018). "Toward a sociological model of Autism." (Doctoral thesis) Available at: https://www.researchgate.net/publication/327318270_ Toward_a_Sociology_of_Autism

TANG, G. et al. (2014). "Loss of mTOR-dependent macroautophagy causes autistic-like synaptic pruning deficits." *Neuron*, no. 83(5), p. 1131-1143.

TOTSIKA, V.; HASTINGS, RP; DUTTON, Y. et al. (2020). "Types and correlates of school non-attendance in students with autism spectrum disorders." *Autism*, no. 24(7), p. 1639-1649.

WEIGELT, S.; KOLDEWYN, K.; KANWISHER, N. (2012). "Face identity recognition in ASD: a review of behavioral studies." *Neuroscience and Biobehavioural Review*, no. 36, p. 1060-1084.

WESTWOOD, H. et al. (2015). "Using Autism-Spectrum Quotient to measure autistic traits in Anorexia Nervosa: a systematic review and meta-analysis." *Journal of Autism and Development Disorders*, no. 46, p. 964-977.

WESTWOOD, H.; MANDY, W.; TCHANTURIA, K. (2017). "Clinical evaluation of autistic symptoms in women with Anorexia Nervosa." *Molecular Autism*, no. 16, p. 812.

WHEELWRIGHT, S. et al. (2010). "Defining the broader, medium and narrow autism phenotype among parents using the Autism Spectrum Quotient (AQ)." *Molecular Autism*, no. 1(1), p. 10-19.

WING, L. (1981). "Asperger's syndrome: a clinical account." *Psychological Medicine*, no. 11(1), p. 115-129.

WING, L.; YEATES, SR; BRIERLEY, LM; GOULD, J. (1976). "The prevalence of early childhood autism: Comparison of administrative and epidemiological studies." *Psychological Medicine*, no. 6(1), p. 89-100.

Pay a visit to:

# Quick Immersion Series

Visit our WEB:
https://www.quickimmersions.com/

You will get:

+Information of all published books

+News of the books in preparation

+You can subscribe to "A Quick Immersion"

+Links to other spaces of our WEB

+Contact us

+Receive timely information on all our titles

This book was translated with a grant from the
*Institut Ramon Llull*

LLLL institut
ramon llull